Acclaim for Dr. Brett Osborn's
Get Serious

"On his own path to self optimization, Dr. Osborn has provided the aspiring body-hacker a battle tested roadmap—with himself, an embodiment of its success."

—Ali R. Malek, MD, FSNIS, Director, Neurointerventional Program and
Comprehensive Stroke Program, St. Mary's Medical Center

*"Dr. Brett Osborn is the real deal. He knows what he's talking about because he lives out the pages of **Get Serious** through his own life, and with his patients, each and every day. The truths he shares about natural health and healing should be shouted from the rooftops. They are even more exciting coming from someone who has earned the respect of the established medical profession. Thank you, Dr. Osborn, for sharing **Get Serious** with the world."*

—Frank King, ND, DC, *The Healing Revolution*

"It takes a brain surgeon to write a no-nonsense, easy-to-understand book on staying fit, smart and healthy at any age."

—Zenon Bilas, *7-time USA Barefoot Waterskiing Champion*

"It's so refreshing to read a book by a neurosurgeon who embraces natural health alternatives.

Dr. Osborn provides science-based advice on exercise, nutrition and diet, along with his specialized knowledge of the brain's role in our overall health. This is a must-read for men and women of all ages!"

—Earl Mindell, RPh, PhD, *Earl Mindell's New Vitamin Bible*

*"This is a serious program, for serious people, with serious schedules, serious families, serious jobs, who want serious results... so, let's **Get Serious**.*

I love Dr. Osborn's no-nonsense approach to fitness and wellness... it's refreshing. In a fitness world that's full of charlatans, with snake oil solvents, Dr. Osborn's method sets the record straight.

Dr. Osborn is a walking billboard for his own program. He lives the lifestyle that he professes, and his book will help you attain your goals safely and swiftly. You shouldn't walk to get this book...you should Sprint !!"

—Jaime Brenkus, *8-minute Abs*

GET
SERIOUS

Dr. Brett Osborn

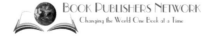

BOOK PUBLISHERS NETWORK
Changing the World One Book at a Time

Book Publishers Network
P.O. Box 2256
Bothell • WA • 98041
Ph • 425-483-3040
www.bookpublishersnetwork.com

10 9 8 7 6 5 4 3 2 1
Printed in the United States of America

LCCN 2014930788
ISBN 978-1-940598-20-8

Editor: Carol Colman
Proofreader: Barbara Kindness
Indexer: Carolyn Acheson
Cover Designer and Typographer: Marsha Slomowitz

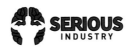

Dedication

To my children
Jack, Ellis and Makenna.

I try to keep up with you every day,
yet I hope (and know)
that you will far surpass me
in every endeavor.

GET SERIOUS

ACKNOWLEDGEMENTS	ix	
FOREWORD	xi	
CHAPTER 1	1	Health: The Choice Is Yours
CHAPTER 2	9	Spending More Money but Getting Sicker
CHAPTER 3	15	Stop Blaming Your Genes
CHAPTER 4	23	Build a Better Body
CHAPTER 5	38	The Pillars: A Step-by-Step Guide
CHAPTER 6	87	Fuel a Better Body
CHAPTER 7	115	Dont Forget Your Brain
CHAPTER 8	125	Supplements 101
CHAPTER 9	143	Keeping Track: At-Home Monitoring
CHAPTER 10	159	Blood Tests to Insist On
CHAPTER 11	167	The Truth about Hormones
APPENDIX	174	The Strength Training Protocol
AFTERWORD	195	
BIBLIOGRAPHY	197	

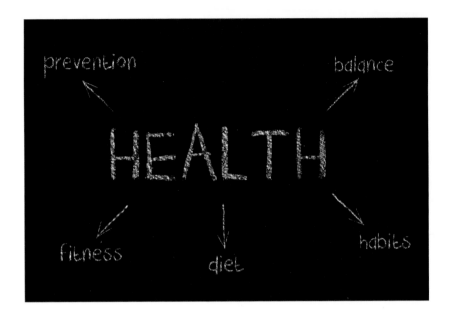

Disclaimer:

The opinions expressed in this book *are not a substitute for qualified medical advice from your personal physician.* Accordingly, *the author assumes no responsibility nor liability* for injury, illness or other malady incurred on account of the information detailed within this manuscript and/or a related website.

Acknowledgements

There's an old saying "Behind every successful man, there is a woman." In the context of this book, my version would read, "Behind every successful man, there are several *brilliant* but even more so, *tolerant* women." I would personally like to thank Carol Colman, editor and author of multiple best-sellers, for helping me focus my thoughts and deliver my best message to the reader. Sheryn Hara and Marsha Slomowitz, I owe much to you both, mainly for putting up with me (and my pedantic nature). What else would you expect from a neurosurgeon? Thank you for making this book so aesthetically appealing. I challenged you to create a "*coffee table book* on health," the first of its kind. And you delivered! Brilliantly. On a similar note I'd like to acknowledge Candace West, photographer, for thinking outside of the box and getting the much-needed (and often unique) shot angles. Marsha Friedman of EMSI, many thanks go out to you for your guidance, unending enthusiasm for your craft and encouragement. *None* of this would have been possible without you. Thank you for facilitating every aspect of this at times daunting task.

Renée Halfhill and Mark Asanovich... Well, just have a look at Chapter 5, the product of your efforts. I am inspired by your passion and relentless pursuit of health. Additional thanks to Jason Neil of Rock Fitness and Doug Johnson of The Zoo for providing me the needed gym space for the photo shoot. Had these two motivated individuals not gone out of their way to accommodate me, readers would have had to "stomach" the dungeon-of-a-garage in which I routinely train. In this context, I'd also like to thank my long-time friend and mentor, David Landau, for his eternal motivation, wealth of exercise knowledge, and 24-hour access to the training facility (or what we refer to as the "lab").

And of course, a big THANK YOU to my family, for your unconditional support, love and insight. You have empowered me. You motivate me to want to make the world a better place. Melissa, thank you for tolerating me during this last year. I am very thankful to have you in my life (particularly for your proofreading skills... just kidding).

That said, I give you the reader (and hopefully *never* a patient), **Get Serious**.

Foreword

The Health & Fitness industry is unregulated. Meaning, absolutely *ANYONE* can practice... whether they are credentialed... *OR NOT!* As such, the Health & Fitness industry is inundated with many practitioners who are well-intended, albeit NOT well educated. This has saturated the market with many fallacious "training" protocols and products that have resulted in a dramatic rise in exercise-related injuries. In a 2010 study published in the *American Journal of Sports Medicine*, it was reported that weight training-related injuries in the United States from 1990 to 2007 increased over 48 percent. Shocking when you consider that the purpose of exercise is to *ENHANCE*... not *ENDANGER* health. The industry is fast becoming one where the blind are leading the blind.

As a practitioner in the Health & Fitness profession for over 30 years, I have served as an NFL Strength & Conditioning Coach for fourteen years, a college Strength & Conditioning Coach for three years, and a high school Strength & Conditioning Coach for twelve years. I have also worked in commercial fitness having managed a Fitness Center for one year. Currently, I am serving as a high school strength coach and speaking nationally on evidence-based strength & conditioning.

As is the case in most of these seminars, the audience is primarily comprised of participants that want to be entertained and are there mainly to receive continuing education units. Occasionally, there are those individuals who are very passionate and have very opinionated beliefs about exercise... that of course they want you to affirm. Rarely do I meet individuals who have actually studied the current exercise science literature. Never have I encountered someone that is passionate about exercise... *and educated about exercise*. That is, until I met Dr. Brett Osborn on one of my speaking tours in West Palm Beach, Florida.

A Board-Certified Neurological Surgeon by trade, Dr. Osborn is passionate about bodybuilding. As you can imagine, I don't encounter too many neurosurgeons that are into bodybuilding. I was intrigued. What I learned about Dr. Osborn's quest for the highly chiseled body was that he coincided his advanced understanding of medicine with his life's search of determining the most productive strength training methodologies. What I also learned was that he wanted to share that knowledge with the world.

Given the limited exercise science acumen of most people, it is easy to understand why so many are readily deceived or misled by the persuasive and clever advertising or charismatic personalities of the "get big now" schemes. Most educators, athletes, parents and fitness consumers are simply unprepared to navigate through the quagmire of exercise misinformation to make informed decisions.

Dr. Osborn's book, **Get Serious**, provides the information to not only objectively cut through the hyperbole, but it will also help to develop an understanding of evidence-based and time-proven principles of prudent, productive, practical and purposeful strength training. Dr. Osborn's easy-to-read, no-nonsense writing style clearly and concisely teaches the basics of exercise, nutrition, dietary supplements, genetics, hormones... and of course, the role of the brain in maximizing training results.

So, if you are looking for a current, mainstream, trendy, fitness "read" that is based on superstition, innuendo, ignorance and a flare for the esoteric, you are in for a surprise! On the other hand, if you are a health enthusiast seeking *REAL RESULTS,* answers to *REAL LIFE* strength training questions, you need to **Get Serious**. If you are an athlete seeking to *MAXIMIZE your performance and MINIMIZE injury*, you need to **Get Serious**. If you are a parent seeking *direction on where to PROFIT most on your INVESTMENT in your children's health*, you need to **Get Serious**. If you are a fitness professional who is appalled with the current state of affairs in commercial exercise today and are looking for an educated and evidence-based methodology, you need to **Get Serious**.

Mark Asanovich, CSCS
Former Strength and Conditioning Coach, NFL

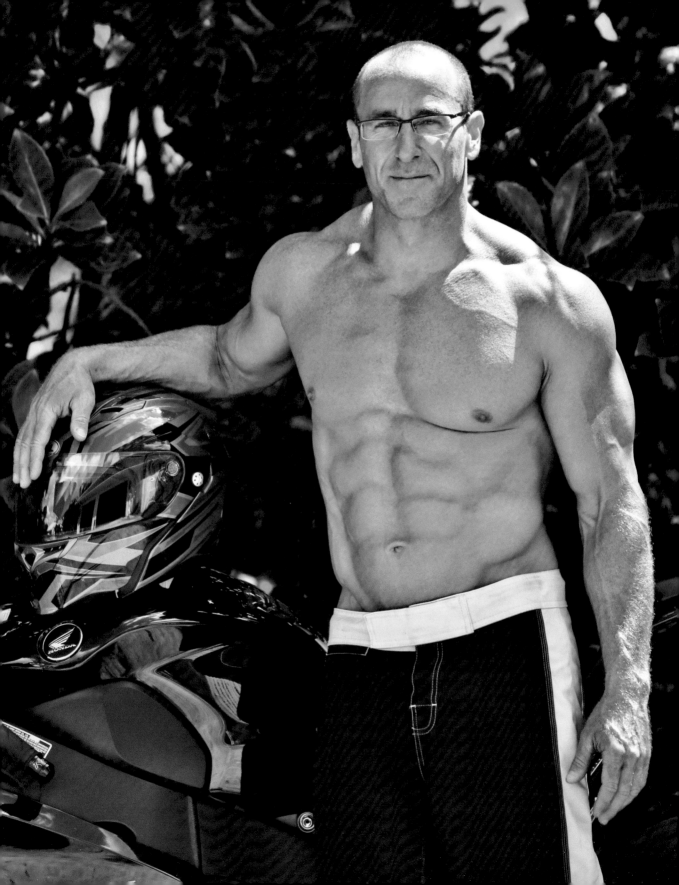

HEALTH
the **CHOICE** is yours

I find myself in an interesting predicament. If people actually followed the advice in this book, my colleagues and I would be performing far fewer operations, ICUs and emergency rooms would have beds to spare, and many hospitals would be forced to shut down because of lack of customers!

And that's fine with me.

I wear two hats. I am a Board-Certified Neurological Surgeon, which means I perform surgery on the brain and spine. I am dually certified in Anti-Aging and Regenerative Medicine. Directing patients to the right lifestyle is an important component of my practice. Although I love performing surgery, I would much rather show people how to stay well—and age well—than have to operate on them after the fact.

I walk the talk. I am also a bodybuilder and have earned a CSCS honorarium from the National Strength and Conditioning Association. I am not the "Do as I say—but not as I do" physician charging you to lose fat and get healthy. It's an embarrassment to the profession that about half of all physicians are either overweight or obese! *I live this life*. Have a look at the pictures. My goal here is to empower you with knowledge to achieve optimal health.

The truth is, *most* ailments of modern-day society are preventable. Yes, most strokes, dementia, heart attack, diabetes, spine disorders, and even most cancers, are *preventable*. I haven't been sick in years, and am in the best physical and mental shape of my life. YOU CAN BE TOO! It's not that difficult, but it does require work and a bit of education. So follow along carefully. Read and **re-read**. Ask questions (I have provided my contact information). And get going! No thinking here. **This is your life, your health. There is nothing more important.**

You wonder, "Why me?"

Too many people spend their lives chasing that hard-earned dollar, investing little time in their own health for "lack of time," only to develop a terminal disease in mid-life. It's too late to stop smoking after you've been diagnosed with lung cancer. The cat is already out of the bag. This disease-oriented approach to health is a reflection of the failed medical system that exists today; one that treats problems after-the-fact. After you've developed that malignant brain tumor or had the heart attack. Then and only then is time of the essence. And the race begins. One's perspective changes. The once unimportant becomes paramount. The word "family" takes on new meaning. You wonder, "Why me?"

Well, why *not* you? What are you doing today to lower your risk for disease? Or are you of the belief that we are simply disease-stricken and lack control? That cancer just occurs? That we are powerless to prevent disease? That our bodies and more specifically our genes run the show? How wrong you are! Are you aware that the vast majority of cancers are preventable?

It's true, diseases don't just happen overnight. Risk factors accumulate as we age, modifiable risk factors. And thankfully they are modifiable, as this gives you control! Those of you with a strong family history of coronary disease, I am talking to you. You are not destined to succumb to a fatal heart attack at age 35! Yes, a positive family history is a risk factor for coronary artery disease, but there are many others. Do you hear me? There are many other modifiable risk factors. **You have ample opportunity to prevent disease.**

And you have the capability! It's time to Get Serious! This book will show you how to preserve your health and save your life. I'll also show you how to vastly improve your life—you'll have more energy, better sex, and be far more productive than you ever thought possible.

When I say that most problems are preventable, I recognize that there are a few unlucky people who have rare genetic problems that we don't yet fully understand. Despite a healthy lifestyle, they may develop a brain tumor or a spinal problem that requires my surgical services. That being said, I have gleaned significant insight into the biomechanics of the human spine by performing a myriad of spinal operations. I can tell you with absolute certainty that most of these people could have prevented their spinal problems if they had only taken care of their bodies when they were younger. And a significant number could solve their problems by taking simple steps, like losing weight and getting more exercise, and eating better. Truth be told, the *vast majority* of spinal ailments can be treated non-operatively. Volumes have been written on just that. Conservative therapies work, period! Why? Because the degenerative process (arthritis) is inflammatory by nature and therefore responds well to exercise and proper nutrition, both of which tend to quell inflammation. Reduced inflammation equates to reduced pain and a slowing of the degenerative process. Get it? And this not only applies to diseases of the spine. Exercise, specifically strength training, and proper nutrition not only serve as discrete *treatment* modalities for various diseases, but also **protect you from disease.**

Well, why *not* you?

This not only applies to diseases of the spine. People who exercise and eat properly live the longest; good habits equate to longevity. There is a huge body of science to back up these assertions, shedding some light on the mechanisms that confer this protective effect. Specifically, as will be discussed later, exercise and good eating habits reduce chemicals naturally produced by the body called "free radicals." The strategies described in this book work by bolstering antioxidants (chemicals that moderate the impact of free radicals), quell inflammation and maintain tight blood sugar control. You may not think of them this way, but *both diet and exercise act as signals to the body,* switching on biochemical processes that ultimately confer protection from a variety of diseases. You will not only become a stronger individual from those sets of resistance training exercises, you will become leaner and healthier. You will get sick less often. You will have more energy; your mood will improve. And it all boils down to biochemistry. Yes, your health is wholly a function of *your individual* biochemistry. And while these complex processes

**RISK FACTORS
FOR DISEASE
THAT REQUIRE NO
SPECIFIC TESTING.**

No needles, nothing.
Poor nutrition, lack
of exercise and
unchecked stress.
Huge players in the
genesis of disease.
And all it takes
to identify these
very modifiable
risk factors is a
little introspection.
Identify first, then
modify. Then do
it again. *Forever.*
Assess, intervene
and then reassess.
You will not only
learn about proper
food choices, but
understand why a
particular food sends
better signals to the
body than another.
And the knowledge
will empower you,
enabling you to
make the right
choice in the future.
Again, the goal here
is *understanding.*

are running in the background 24/7, on autopilot if you will, you still have a great degree of control. You can intervene and steer the ship by providing the proper signals. By making the right choices. You have to choose to be healthy.

Yes, **health is a choice. It is not a right.** If I can teach you one thing, it is that. No one owes you anything. **Your health is a privilege and you must earn it.** It takes effort on your behalf. Do not expect your doctor to *provide* you with health. Sadly, this notion of entitlement pervades the younger generation. Well I've got news for you, health is not for the entitled. Don't believe me? Just check the statistics. Inactivity rates are on the rise. There is an obesity epidemic. People are disease stricken at younger and younger ages. Why? Poor choices, *not* poor doctors.

YOU must take an active role in your own health by first assuming responsibility for your actions and their potential consequences. Don't sue McDonald's for **your** obesity. Don't blame Philip Morris for **your** being stricken with lung cancer. **YOU** are in control, no one else.

You have the capacity to attain good health.

And that is my charge to you. You have the capacity to attain good health. It's easier than you think but nevertheless takes work. The problem today lies in the fact that there is too much interference. Between the internet (*mis*information superhighway) and magazines showcasing the latest and greatest trends in nutrition and physical fitness, consumers have difficulty differentiating between fact and fiction. Low carbohydrate diet? Low fat diet? Which is it? And why? Machine-based, Nautilus-style training or free-weights? Google any of these topics. Rest assured you will find thousands of sites touting the merits of each, leaving you more confused. So where do you turn? Not to another website. These are some of the worst sources of medical information. Instead get *back to basics*. Educate yourself. Strive to understand exercise and nutrition basics. This book will help you. *You must come to grips with the fact that our current healthcare system fosters disease not health.* Protect yourself from the system by arming yourself with knowledge. Become an informed patient and an informed trainee. Take matters into your own hands.

How? First, by identifying risk factors for disease and then modifying them. Like I said before, one isn't disease-free one day and the next admitted to a hospital with a fatal brain hemorrhage. Typically, such strokes are the result of poorly controlled hypertension. Elevated blood pressure is a risk factor for stroke. A *modifiable* risk factor. And that diagnosis can be made from the comforts of your home. Go buy a blood pressure cuff! And what about your blood sugar? Are you "insulin resistant?" If you're obese, you likely have insulin resistance. Unto itself, obesity is a risk factor for many diseases including cancer. Why? For one thing, obesity-associated *inflammation* primes the system for the development of age-related diseases, many of which will flat-out kill you. Is this you? Do you meet the criteria to be considered obese? What other disease risk factors do you have? It's likely that you don't *know* of any (which certainly does not equate to health). No problem. We're going to fix that.

Take matters into your own hands.

In this book you will learn about the multitude of disease risk factors such as insulin resistance, dyslipidemia, obesity, hypertension (cumulatively known as Metabolic Syndrome), hormonal imbalance, and the role of chronic inflammation in the genesis of disease. More importantly you will come to understand their interrelationship, how many of the *disease processes themselves* are interrelated, and how the presence of one may foster development of another. Remember, you're not one day stricken with type II diabetes. It creeps up on you. But not if you catch it first!

By testing for these risk factors, you will be able to identify them if and when they rear their ugly heads. But don't wait until you develop florid symptoms of disease *prior to testing*. Test now! I can assure you that you will identify risk factors that were flying beneath the radar. A low vitamin D_3 level for example. That's a risk factor for disease. With a small amount of effort (taking a single supplement capsule daily), you can dramatically reduce your chances of developing certain diseases, breast cancer for example. A simple intervention albeit one with high impact.

The same goes for exercise. It is critical for us to exercise on a daily basis. Lack of exercise predisposes us to disease. Our bodies are meant

LONGEVITY

HEALTH

EXERCISE

Wellness road

NUTRITION

REST

POSITIVE THINKING

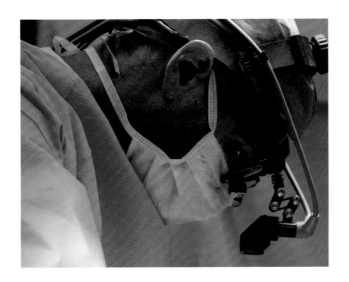

As a neurosurgeon, I am faced with daily stresses. Unchecked stress results in poor performance, but more importantly unchecked stress is deleterious to your health. It is difficult to quantify. You can't see it. It is an intangible.

to move. We are designed to exercise or should I say **engineered?** We are, at base level, machines with operating instructions written in code, the genetic code. Exercise switches on those particular genes associated with health and longevity. The right type of exercise confers protection from disease. Yes, it augments your immunity! You will be a leaner, sharper and healthier individual as a result of exercise. So don't even *think* you are exempt from exercise because you "have no medical problems." You will, in time. That said, *the lack of exercise is a risk factor for disease. Inactivity is a risk factor for disease*, period. And you have no excuses. Make exercise a priority! If I can exercise with my very busy schedule, so can you.

As a neurosurgeon, I am faced with daily stresses to which I have become accustomed. This took practice and mental fortitude (more so than the technical aspects of surgery demanded). Unchecked stress results in poor performance, but more importantly unchecked stress is deleterious to your health. Until recently, this was underappreciated. Why? It is difficult to quantify. You can't see it. It is an intangible. But it has the capacity to literally decimate your health.

Psychological stressors on a chronic basis initiate cascades of hormonal responses which ultimately serve a catabolic effect—that is, it eats up your muscle. Body weight will fluctuate, muscle mass will decline, blood glucose elevation will promote the development of insulin resistance and potentially the Metabolic Syndrome. This primes the system for age-related disease such as atherosclerotic heart disease or "clogging of the arteries." Am I telling you that chronic stress is associated with coronary artery disease? Damn right. And it can kill you dead in even smaller doses than once thought.

Have you ever heard of "voodoo" death? It is a well-documented phenomenon in fact. *Inexplicable* deaths have been reported among Australian natives who had been cursed by tribal witch doctors or had a "bone pointed at them." Dr. Walter Cannon, credited with describing this phenomenon in 1942, postulates that a "***persistent*** and profound emotional state may induce a disastrous fall of blood pressure, ending in death. Lack of food and drink would collaborate with the damaging emotional effects, to induce the fatal outcome." This effect is believed to be due to overactivation of the "sympathetic" system, the division of our nervous system which in part is related to the "flight or fight response," our stress response. You know, the one that is activated when the lion is chasing you? That one. My point? ***Chronic*** stress is extremely detrimental to your health and must be tempered. Identify those things that "stress you out" and take the necessary steps to maintain them at bay. You are in control! Do not allow stress to reign unchecked. Stop it dead in its tracks before it evolves into a chronic problem and compromises your health.

Easy? Yes. But it requires a little know-how and commitment. The knowledge, I hope to give you in this book. The commitment? That I leave to you. Health is a lifestyle. It's a choice. There are no shortcuts. Fad diets or trendy "12 weeks to a great body" exercise programs do not lead to permanent, sustainable change. ***There is only one solution: a persistent effort to maintain health and thereby prevent disease.*** Too many people out there are seeking the latest and greatest in fitness and nutrition regimens, ever-searching for that elixir. They are attracted to a new technique or a new technology, but in reality, there is *nothing* new. There is simply more interference. The body functions physiologically in the same manner it did 10,000 years ago! It can't be tricked. Successful weight loss regimens are simply permutations of the **same** principles applied to human physiology. There are no "secrets." Stick to the basics, the fundamentals, as detailed in this book. It's your safest bet for long-lasting health.

YOU ARE IN CONTROL. Now **Get Serious** and get going...

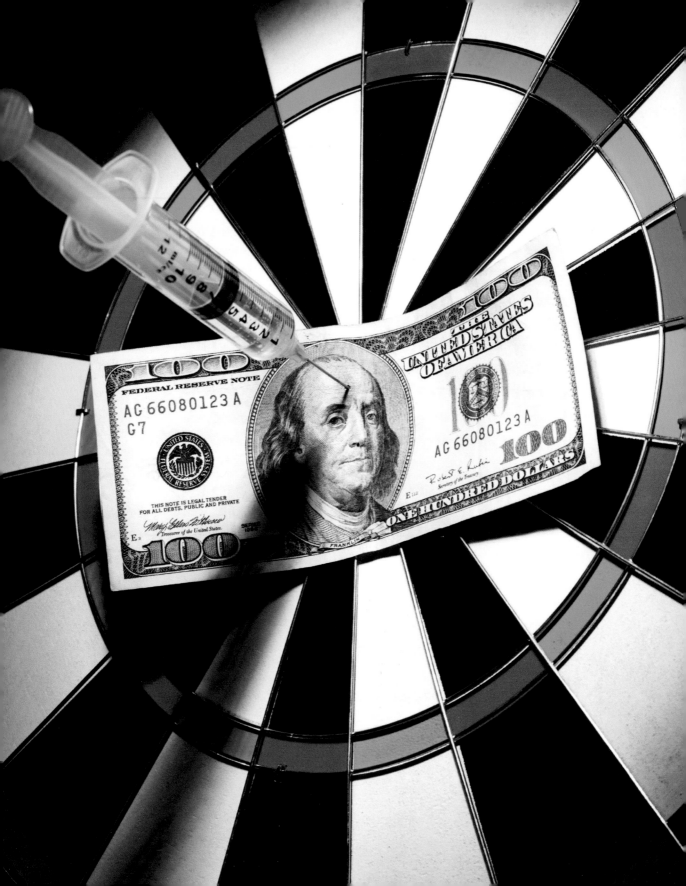

2 SPENDING

more money but getting SICKER

Did you ever run up a "down" escalator when you were a kid? You ran and ran, faster and faster, but despite your best efforts, you ended up going backwards. Truly an "uphill battle!"

Unfortunately a similar phenomenon is occurring today. Technology is advancing at a breakneck pace, we know more and more about the genesis of disease, yet health burden rises. We are fatter than ever. The incidence of type II diabetes has skyrocketed. Healthcare costs have risen in parallel. What the hell is going on? Logic suggests the opposite should be occurring, but there is nothing logical about healthcare, as you will see.

We are smarter now than ever before. We are armed with data to battle disease on the front line. And we do this, fairly well in fact. *Once these diseases surface*, the war begins, with full engagement of the enemy, *but not before.*

Yes, we are extremely skilled at keeping people alive *once they are disease-stricken*. Is that the goal, an "after-the-fact" approach that positions people behind the eight ball once risk factors have accumulated and disease sets in? So why has this strategy been fostered not only here but worldwide? Some of it stems from tradition: identify the signs and symptoms of disease, establish the diagnosis and *then* treat. While this is a logical method, it is flawed. At base level, it is simply well... *wrong*.

What has to be realized early on is that each one of us is stricken with a disease in our late 20's to early 30's, one that essentially primes the playing field for other health problems. It is the disease of **aging**. You may be thinking, "aging is not a disease." Well, if it's not, why does this *non*-disease kill 100,000 people per day? *Two-thirds* of the death toll worldwide is due to age-related disease. So what is considered an age-related disease? Let's see... cancer, diabetes, heart disease and Alzheimer's disease. *All are age-related diseases*.

Problem #1 therefore stems from an *overt lack of education*. Did you know that the vast majority of cancers are environmental and therefore potentially preventable? They are not at base level due to genetic defects as was once thought. (More on this later.) Type II diabetes? Preventable. Heart disease too. The treatment of heart disease is *neither* bypass surgery nor angioplasty. In fact, these procedures have fallen under much scrutiny recently. Similarly, the treatment for Alzheimer's disease is *neither* Namenda nor Aricept. It is prevention. Enter problem #2.

Money. The population is aging and acquiring disease, preventable disease, right? In the case of Alzheimer's disease, the most common form of dementia, patients are prescribed medications like Namenda and Aricept. The disease invariably progresses and with good intention, doctors prescribe additional medication. Money by the boatload is dumped into Big Pharma's coffers. Reeling in the loot, pharmaceutical companies are de-incentivized to find a "cure" for aging or age-related disease. It's akin to shooting themselves in the foot.

Keep in mind too that the above drugs are only modestly effective in treating the symptoms of Alzheimer's disease. Yet we continue to treat the symptoms not the disease process itself, to the chagrin of Big Pharma. Remember, **there is money in disease not health.** Don't believe me? Take a look at the efficacy of some of the cancer "treatments" offered today. What a joke! One has to wonder who is benefiting. Patients? Think again... Big Pharma. Drug trial data are often skewed, statistically manipulated, to demonstrate efficacy of chemotherapies and downplay side effects (Vioxx anyone?). Billions of research dollars are at stake should the trials fail. Are you hearing me?

And what efforts have the pharmaceutical companies made to *prevent* disease as opposed to treating it? Few, relatively speaking. They profit from the sick, get it? Big Pharma's apathy may also be secondary to the limited insurance reimbursements for preventive therapies. Short-term, reimbursing for preventive medications would be a fiscal loss to HMO's and PPO alike; long-term, however, this would save many lives and a mint's worth of money. The CEO's of said companies only seek the *immediate* capital gains however. Stockholders are pleased, yet plan members, people, you, are disease-stricken.

And herein lies the irony. Are the CEOs of these large insurance companies truly aware of the yearly dollars squandered on percutaneous coronary intervention procedures or "cardiac caths"? Yes, *squandered*. There is little data to support the, at times, irrational practice of angioplasty, stent and coronary bypass surgeries. In fact the Courage Trial, a major 2007 study, demonstrated that in patients with known coronary disease, there is little if any difference in deaths, heart attacks or strokes between those with optimal medical treatment and those undergoing percutaneous procedures. This reinforces the latest science that heart attacks are *not* due to stenotic (narrowed) arteries but due to acute clot formation on existing atherosclerotic plaque. Otherwise, interventional procedures (that open narrowed arteries) would significantly reduce the incidence of coronary events. But this is not the case! Patients fare *equally well* with optimal medical therapy.

So why the tremendous overuse of angioplasty/stent and bypass procedures? Guess… Money! Annual reimbursements to both doctor and hospital for said procedures approximate $50 billion. And nearly 70 percent of these procedures are unnecessary. A far more effective "treatment" strategy would place emphasis on preventive modalities: exercise, sound nutrition, stress reduction and medical optimization. Cardiologists should be reimbursed handsomely for preventing heart attacks, not treating them. That's a radical thought!

One of the goals of this book is to arm you with the knowledge to thrive within this failed healthcare system. What do I mean? The current system fosters and perpetuates disease as opposed to health. At base level, there is a stark lack of knowledge, outright ignorance, if you will, of nutrition and the body's requirement for *daily* exercise. And it's our fault! Healthcare professionals and teachers are still losing this battle as educators. This is evidenced by the rising obesity rates (30 percent of adults are obese). *Childhood* obesity rates have skyrocketed (many thanks to the video game manufacturers). This translates into early onset diabetes and the Metabolic Syndrome (described later as a syndrome with a high associated risk for heart attack and stroke).

Physical education in school systems is *de*-emphasized. What ever happened to the Presidential Fitness Awards? Kids nowadays actually believe that they are exercising using Wii Fit. And parents have been similarly hoodwinked. Any way you skin it, there is absolutely no way that a child is getting enough physical activity to effectively prevent disease. Health classes should be a mandatory, integral part of *every* child's curriculum, taken *every* year beginning in elementary school. Ideally, there would also be baseline standards of physical fitness for boys and girls alike, period. And these should be to some degree challenging.

The effects of these physical requirements are far-reaching. Once an individual incorporates exercise into his daily regimen, it becomes an integral part of his or her life. There simply is no better preventive strategy especially if such "physicality" is coupled with sound diet and nutrition. And the data suggests just that, as noted by the title of this study, "Higher moderate-to-vigorous-intensity physical activity (MVPA) time by children and adolescents was associated with better cardiometabolic risk factors regardless of the amount of sedentary time." (JAMA, February 15, 2012-Vol 307, No. 7) **Exercise is protective of the body.** Say it: "Exercise is protective of the body." Let me make it simple, get your kids off their asses if you truly want to make an impact on their health, now and in the future.

Similarly, guide your children's food choices. Teach them the bad as well as the good. They should understand at an early age that a Big Mac provides little, if any, nutritional benefit and that fast food is not a household staple. As will be discussed later, even an "optimized" diet fails to render all the nutrients required for optimal health. This is becoming ever more obvious. Take, for example, vitamin D_3. The 100 i.u. of Vitamin D_3 found in a glass of fortified milk is a laughable quantity (as is the RDA by the way). And no, you are likely not getting enough sunlight to make up the dietary deficit. Vitamin D_3 deficiency is rampant. And insufficient vitamin D_3 is linked to many age-related disorders including cancer, vascular disease and osteoporosis. Therefore, supplements are a necessary component of our daily nutritional intake. And this must begin at an early age. **Prevent problems before they begin.**

Keep in mind too that you cannot rely on the pharmaceutical industry to educate you as to the merits of nutritional supplementation. It is simply not in their best interest. Supplements are considered "food" to the FDA and therefore cannot be patented. Without patent protection, supplements cannot be exclusively produced by a single pharmaceutical company. No monopoly on the market equates to limited profits; and limited profits equates to limited interest in producing such products. By virtue of this, pharmaceutical companies generate far more dollars from the ill-stricken as opposed to the healthy. Why? Because the vast majority of these individuals are on multiple drugs to treat their chronic diseases. And guess what, we're living longer *with* those chronic diseases!

So this self-perpetuating cycle needs to be teased apart, the details elucidated and stop-gap measures instituted by YOU, because let's face it, the healthcare system *will not* save you. Socialized medicine, if instituted, will not rectify this situation either. Yes, everyone will theoretically have access to care, but the quality of that care is questionable. Doctors' practices will be further diluted by the patient onslaught. Less time per patient equates to less comprehensive care. And preventive medicine will become an even less important focus of doctors' practices. The health burden will continue to escalate in this country. People are living longer, accumulating disease and simply existing in a decrepit state until their demise. Nursing homes and long-term care facilities are occupied by products of the failed healthcare environment. Such patients, those with one or more chronic conditions, account for 84 percent of all healthcare spending. They are the heaviest users of healthcare services and a sump for Medicare dollars. And we are all aware of the challenges that Medicare faces *at this point*, let alone in 10 years when the aged population has grown in size. The program will be bankrupt by then in fact, according to calculations. Extrapolating, what ultimately will "do-in Medicare" (mismanagement aside) is the population suffering from chronic age-related diseases. Preventable disease! And don't expect your doctor to save you.

The goal of this book is to educate you the consumer, the patient, and allow you to assume care of your own health. Take charge and you will be able to assist your physician as he/she strives to provide optimal care for you. Ultimately, this will allow you to live a healthier, longer and productive life.

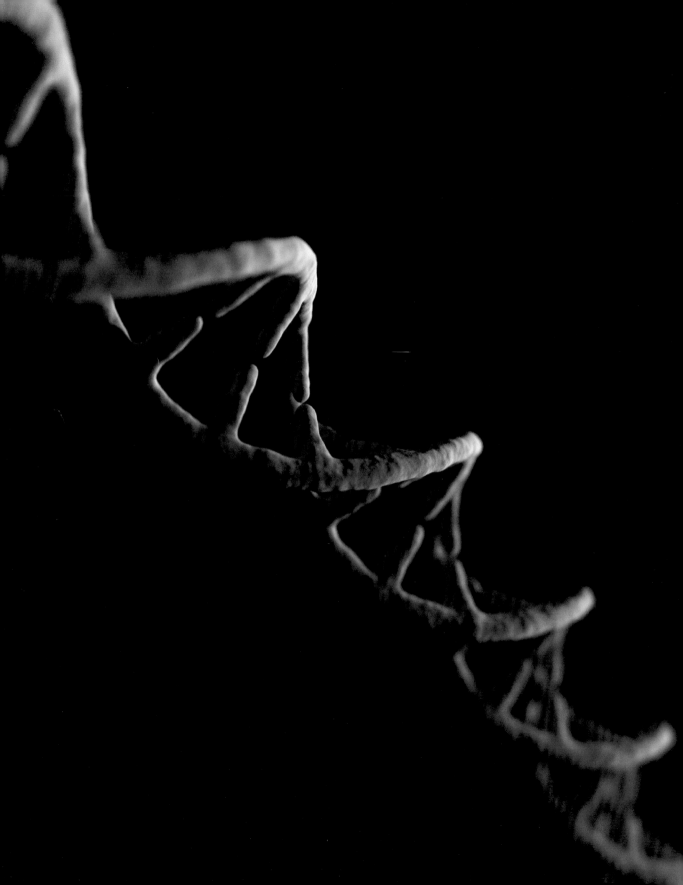

3

BLAMING

your genes

This book is about YOU taking control of the things that you can to live the longest, healthiest life possible. That means following an optimal diet, doing the right workout, and taking supplements that help keep you well. And yet, I'm sure many of you believe that despite all your good intentions and hard work, you will be sabotaged by "bad genes."

I hear this every day from my patients, especially those who come to me with low-back pain, a very common problem. They are under the misconception that spinal fusion surgery will somehow magically relieve their pain. Many of these patients are obese. (Get it? Back pain? Lugging around 20-100 pounds of excess fat? See the connection?) After 1,000+ spine operations under my belt, I can still provide little if any help *as a surgeon* except in the select few. Surgery for low-back pain in isolation is, for the most part, a no-no as outcomes historically are poor. Instead we should be looking inside *ourselves*.

Patients are taken aback when I begin the diatribe.

"What do you mean a fusion operation won't help my back?" is the standard response. "You're saying that I have to lose weight?"

"Yes, you have to lose weight and begin exercising to strengthen your back."

"But exercising hurts my back and I can't lose weight because *everyone in my family is fat. I have fat genes.*"

Aha! The fault lies with their genes. The fact that they are sedentary 99 percent of the time and eat a horrible diet has nothing to do with it.

Of course, this is a pathetic excuse. It's as if these individuals are condemned to a life of obesity by virtue of their genetic makeup. That is simply not true for all but a tiny minority. GET SERIOUS people! While you certainly are a product of your genes, by no means are you being victimized by your DNA. **You** *are ultimately in control.* So stop blaming your genes! Keep in mind that the *majority* of diseases (barring those of a congenital nature) are environmental in origin. Yes, this even includes cancer!

It was previously thought that if one developed cancer, he or she "had bad genes." Cancer was "genetic." Bullshit. *Cancer is an environmental disease,* period. As many as 90-95 percent of all types of cancers have their roots in the environment and lifestyle. As noted in a study published in *Pharmacology Research*, a respected, mainstream medical journal, "The evidence indicates that of all cancer-related deaths, almost 25–30 percent are due to tobacco, as many as 30–35 percent are linked to diet, about 15–20 percent are due to infections, and the remaining percentage are due to other factors like radiation, stress, physical activity, environmental pollutants, etc."

This is good news! Why? Because *you* have the power and the ability to alter your health for the better. There is no pre-determinism; you are not destined to be disease-stricken. **You and you alone have a choice, a choice to be healthy or sick.** And this choice is independent of the hand your parents dealt you.

But wait a minute, there has got to be some merit to this gene stuff, right? Angelina Jolie recently had a prophylactic double mastectomy based upon the results of her genetic testing. What gives? Well, here's the deal. There are *specific* genes which if mutated are associated with the development of certain cancers (BRCA1 and BRCA2 in the context of breast cancer). *If* high-risk individuals harboring these mutations were identified, they potentially could intervene early, thereby preventing disease. In this particular subset of patients, genetic testing *in retrospect* has proven very worthwhile and potentially lifesaving. Keep in mind, however, that the incidence of the BRCA mutation in the general population is *low*. And as a woman, you are ***much*** more likely to die of another disease that has a genetic component: atherosclerotic heart disease or coronary artery disease. Yes, according to the American Heart Association, heart disease claims nearly 500,000 women yearly.

This is nearly **12** times more than reported breast-cancer related deaths in 2009! (Source: Centers for Disease Control) Accordingly, educating the public about *this* preventable disease should be more the focus of our attention than radical celebrity-endorsed procedures that will benefit relatively few, specifically those with *the gene*.

What is DNA?

So what are these "genes" anyway? Let's start with a more basic question. What is DNA? Well, deoxyribonucleic acid or DNA is the inheritable, self-replicating material that contains all of the information necessary to build and maintain an organism, like a human being. And get this, *each* cell in your body has all the necessary genetic instructions (within coiled chromosomal DNA) to rebuild your *entire* body. Remember Dolly the cloned sheep? She was living proof of this concept. So could a human be cloned? Of course. Do you know any identical twins? Clones! This type of cloning is a natural occurrence in contrast to the two commonly discussed types of human cloning: *therapeutic* and *reproductive* cloning (Source: *Wikipedia*). Specific details aside, cloning is simply "the process of creating an exact copy of a biological unit from which it was derived." (Source: Biology-Online.org) This is *only* possible because the genetic code (that which is written into your DNA) and more specifically its interpretation within *each* bodily cell is preserved. Huh? Yes, all of your cells possess the machinery to uncoil chromosomal DNA, interpret the instructions and generate gene products (for example, proteins) *according to those instructions*. This cellular language is preserved, human to human. We *all* speak it. At least our cells do. Harvested DNA from an organism can therefore be "transplanted" into an empty egg cell and voilà, a clone is born.

DNA across a particular species is static. *Homo sapiens (human beings)*, the last surviving species of the genus *homo,* have a predictable, conserved genetic code. Your DNA is organized in a nearly identical manner to that of your neighbor and in fact very similarly to that of our closest primate relative with only 1.2 percent inter-species divergence. But what drove the evolutionary process from our common ancestor? Our forebrains enlarged in parallel with our reasoning capacity yet our physical strengths declined relative to that of the great apes. These changes are undoubtedly the result of selective environmental pressures which gradually mutated the genome in a multi-step process. Our "humanness" is the result of an evolutionary process with adaptations suited to our modern world. Brawn has been exchanged for brains as we no longer hunt or forage as means of survival. No longer do we climb trees and harvest our own fruit. We walk upright. And while we still have our tail*bones*, we've lost our tails! Why? Selective "pressures" have stimulated change at a *genetic* level over hundreds of thousands of years.

These changes are not those responsible for variations in eye color for example, but for gross changes, species-specific changes, that are responsible for facial shape or a specific contractile protein in muscle. These species-specific characteristics cannot be altered over a short time course. They are too "hard-wired" into one's genome. For example, a *human* produces a *specific* set of inflammatory proteins in response to an injury. These proteins are products of *our* genes. And while some may be shared with chimpanzees by virtue of our genetic similarities, it is likely that a starfish possesses entirely different inflammatory mediators: those of a *starfish*. And these are immutable. Their molecular makeup is conserved across the species.

Whether or not these chemicals are present in the serum *at any instant in time*, however, is a function of the environment *at that particular instant.* This is an acute process. Genes aren't being altered as during an evolutionary (or devolutionary) process; their *products* are simply being expressed. Proteins are being assembled as the genes are being "translated" within the cell. But what "turns a gene on," ordering the cell (say a liver cell or hepatocyte) to produce and secrete a *specific* protein? The answer: various *environmental* stimuli. And there are myriads of them. From the presence of bacteria within the bloodstream to a change in bodily temperature or a direct hormone-gene interaction—all affect expression of a particular and likely a set of genes. Therefore, genes may be switched "on" and "off." To complicate matters, some genes control the expression of others.

So why is this important? Why am I telling you this? Because optimal health is associated with optimal gene expression. **And you are in control, not the genes!**

Cancer, as we discussed, is for the most part an environmental disease. We are "showing" our genes the wrong stimuli, exposing our DNA to environmental toxins (in many forms) and guess what? Mutations form. Mutations in *tumor suppressor* genes. These protective genes normally function in a variety of ways to assure that cells with mutated DNA (from a spontaneous event, UV radiation, etc.) do not divide or reproduce. But when *these* suppressor genes are mutated, our cells have in essence lost their guardians. Mutations in the p53 suppressor gene, for example, are associated with various types of cancers, namely breast, colorectal, liver, lung, and ovarian cancers.

As a neurosurgeon, I often treat the lethal brain cancer known as glioblastoma multiforme, also associated with a p53 mutation. Sadly, by the time these

> *I often treat the lethal brain cancer known as glioblastoma multiforme, associated with a p53 mutation. By the time patients present with symptoms, their very aggressive tumors have infiltrated large areas of the brain. It is of utmost importance therefore that we detect such tumors earlier or better yet, prevent them.*

patients present to the hospital with symptoms such as headache and weakness, their very aggressive tumors have infiltrated large areas of the brain, limiting the efficacy of even the best treatment options. It is of utmost importance therefore that we detect such tumors earlier or better yet, *prevent* them, in light of their environmental origin. Easier said than done, unfortunately. It takes just a single cancer cell to slip through the body's robust surveillance system and wreak havoc.

This being the case, how do we combat such a disease? Can we, given its complexity? Or should we be looking at the bigger picture, lumping together all of the most lethal diseases and searching for a common cause? The answer is a resounding **YES!** In recent years, *inflammation* has come to the forefront as a major player in the genesis of atherosclerotic heart disease, cerebrovascular disease, diabetes and cancer. From my standpoint, *all diseases have an inflammatory component, all of them.* And this is where we should focus our efforts *primarily*, from a preventive standpoint. Hunting down genetic mutations in *existing* tumors is too late. Instead we should be *preventing* the genetic mutations and protecting the genome by limiting free radical production and reducing oxidative stress. This will ultimately reduce the incidence of *all* diseases, not just cancer, as most have similar origins. Does it surprise you that Alzheimer's disease is referred to as "type *III* diabetes" by virtue of their similar pathophysiology? It shouldn't. Nor should the preventable nature of these diseases.

So how does one not only protect their cells and by virtue their genes, but also utilize their genes to optimize health? Remember, genes are capable of being turned on and off like switches in response to various environmental stimuli. Ideally, those genes integral to the induction and maintenance of bodily inflammation should be switched on *transiently*, for example in the context of a bacterial invader. We develop a fever in response to the gene product TNF-α (tumor necrosis factor-alpha) and IL-6 (interleukin-6). These cytokines or cellular messengers stimulate the host's immune system to mount a response against the bacterial pathogen in an effort to clear it from the body. Here's the problem. *Chronic* exposure to these inflammatory gene products is associated with a variety of diseases, namely those that kill the majority of Americans.

Restated, *acute* inflammation is protective of the body. It is integral to our immune response, wound healing and repair (with or without hypertrophy) of exercise-induced muscle damage. Without inflammation, our workouts would be fruitless, inducing little if any growth. We simply would never build those stronger muscles nor a better body. *Chronic* inflammation on the other hand serves absolutely no benefit. On the contrary, it *is only detrimental*.

Unfortunately, in many of us, this flame burns unchecked and disease accumulates. Blame no one except yourself and certainly not your genes. You are "insulting" your genes by presenting them with bad stimuli such as poor nutrition, tobacco smoke and a lack of exercise. You'd take offense if someone insulted you, right? Well, their response to these environmental threats is the initiation (and perpetuation) of an inflammatory response. The associated collateral damage is manifested as disease, potentially preventable disease. And this includes cancer!

There are really no good or bad genes: the trick is turning on the right genes at the right time. Nuclear factor-$\kappa\beta$ or NF-$\kappa\beta$, for example, has been implicated in tumorigenesis (the formation of cancer) but is integral to cellular responses to stimuli such as stress, cytokines, free radicals, ultraviolet irradiation, oxidized LDL, and bacterial or viral antigens. Sounds like a double-edged sword, doesn't it? Without the help of NF-$\kappa\beta$, we would be unable to mount an inflammatory response and defend ourselves from the constant onslaught of bacterial and viral invaders. Dysregulation of this inflammatory process is disastrous, however. So how does one ride the fine line between too much and too little? It's merely a matter of providing your body with proper stimulation, in essence "showing your genes" the right stuff and concomitantly shielding them from the bad. Unfortunately, in an increasing number of individuals, the bad outweighs the good: inflammation runs rampant, free radical burden is high and defenses are down. Disease escalates. And it is *our* fault, a direct result of poor exercise habits (laziness), toxin exposure and poor nutrition.

SO STOP BLAMING YOUR GENES.
TAKE CONTROL.

The emerging field of epigenetics, which includes nutrigenomics, addresses just how our food interacts with and affects our genes. The food you eat, for example, specifically its micro and macro-nutrient composition, can markedly affect the activity of genes, as demonstrated in a landmark study published in the Proceedings of the National Academy of Sciences. Dr. Dean Ornish and his research team demonstrated that lifestyle modifications such as a low-fat, whole food, plant-based diet modulate gene expression in the prostate gland. The down-regulated genes are associated with chronic diseases such as type II diabetes, obesity and even cancer, potentially explaining the protective effect of intensive lifestyle modification on disease incidence. Similarly, resistance training has been shown to have beneficial effects on one's *genome*. Gene expression is clearly modulated by rigorous strength training. Such up-and-down regulation is not limited to muscular-specific genes but also to those governing the *aging* process! It is not serendipitous that those engaged in a well-designed strength training program "appear" to cling to their youth for longer periods. Sedentary onlookers may assume that "she just has good genes." In the context of the above, however, it may be better stated that "she just has *turned on* the good genes." Of 596 genes associated with age in physiologically normal individuals, those 179 that were associated with *both* aging and exercise showed a marked reversal to youthful levels after a six-month resistance training regimen, according to the study.

A sedentary lifestyle and poor diet can force our genes to behave in a manner that is detrimental to our health; similarly, excess stress is another toxin that can work against us. Do you ever feel that you need a week off from work? You should probably request one. Psychological stressors on a chronic basis initiate cascades of genetically-mediated responses that have deleterious effects on the body. Simply put, it's bad for you. Body weight fluctuates, muscle mass declines, and blood glucose skyrockets promoting the development of insulin resistance (IR) and the Metabolic Syndrome. As a result, your immune system is compromised and disease sets in.

Unfortunately, many Americans are making poor lifestyle choices. We are the second-fattest country in the world despite having the easiest access to gyms and fitness facilities. We are sending our genes the wrong messages. Not unexpectedly, chronic diseases run rampant. **I challenge each and every one of you to take control.** Your genes are *yours*. You own them, not the other way around. So don't blame them for your ailments. Instead use them as a stepping stone to optimal health. After all, they've evolved along with us to facilitate our survival, not impede it, right?

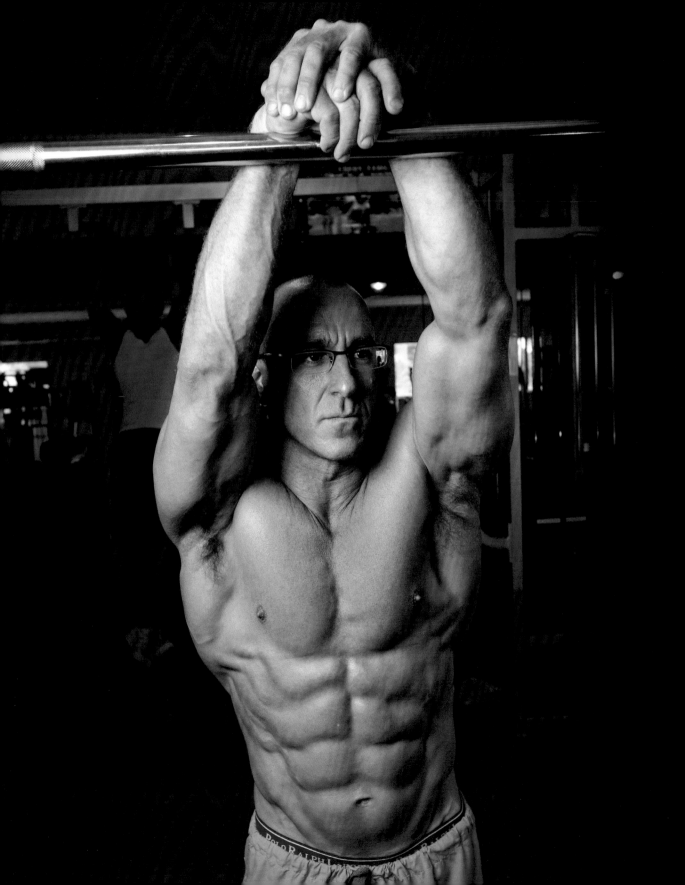

4

BUILD a better BODY

Our bodies are designed to do hard physical work, but our modern, mechanized society has robbed us of the opportunities to do this in our everyday lives.

The environmental stressors that drove muscular development in the era of cave men and women, for example, do not exist today. No skulking tigers in search of human prey that forced us to fight or flee on a moment's notice. Nor do civilized humans have to hunt for survival armed with only the most primitive of tools. Modern day "challenges" take the form of training facilities geared towards harnessing the human potential. We call them "gyms." (In most cases, I call them "worthless.")

The primal setting under which our ancestors thrived has been transformed into airy, high tech arenas touting scantily clad women, a dazzling array of machines that often do much of the work for you, and a corporate brand. Good intentions aside, this is rarely conducive to proper strength training which, in truth, requires little more than a set of weights and a few basic exercises.

It's that simple. (See Chapter 5) Instead, gyms try to outdo each other by offering technologies and gimmicks that generate memberships, like elliptical machines, Stairmasters™, and hybrid classes (e.g. Zumba®), which may be fun but deliver minimal benefit often at the expense of skeletal muscle. This is the primary reason why the vast majority of gym-goers fail to achieve any of their physical goals year after year. Climbing 15,000 flights of rotating stairs is not going to get you very far in terms of creating a stronger, better body.

In contrast, the strength enhancement from the application of a *proper* strength training regimen will improve your life outside the gym. Your golf or tennis game will improve. Likely you will run faster. Concomitantly, your mental acuity and focus will sharpen as the data suggests. You will have more stamina to get through the day and you will sleep better at night. This is as true for women as it is for men.

So regardless of your gender or age, your workout goal should be to get stronger.

Continued progress is essential for health maintenance and well within your capabilities, despite your age. I repeat, **age has nothing to do with it.** You work to achieve *your* full potential. Sure, a 20-year-old may perform better than an 80-year-old, but I recently read about a 91-year-old weightlifting champion who could lift a 187.2 pound metal bar over his chest! I'm not telling you this because I expect you to perform the same feats, but merely to encourage you to open your mind and not set any artificial barriers to what you can do. With proper training undergone in a consistent manner, you will find yourself getting stronger with each workout.

To the layperson, strength is the often desired, hard to reach physical power claimed by the select. The term itself conjures up images of Herculean figures hovering over heaps of weights for hours on end. It's completely wrong: such toilsome labor is unnecessary and such practices inefficient! Strength and the ultimate development of a lean, sleek physique may be attained with a properly prescribed strength-training regimen in less than 3-4 hours per week. Training more may in fact prove detrimental and act as an impediment to progress.

There is a simpler, less time consuming, more effective way to work out and get the results that you want. Once you understand how we make muscle, you will see why so much of what is done in modern gyms is a waste of time.

The only way to develop strength and build muscle is to progressively overload a muscle group through proper exercise. That means working the muscle to its full potential. It takes hard work, and it doesn't happen overnight. Initially, strength will be realized in the improved ability of an individual's performance in a particular movement or exercise. Weight loads may increase, as will the rep count, however there may be no accompanying *physical* change. In other words, a man who is looking to create bigger biceps may not see any real increase in size initially; similarly, a woman who is striving for sculpted Madonna arms may not get there immediately. Don't become discouraged; this is normal! Positive changes are happening! You just can't quite see them yet. What has occurred is an improvement in neuromuscular efficiency, the so-called "learning effect."

As an adaptive response to the imposed stress, the body is making efforts to compensate *first* by improving the pattern of muscular activation (also known as recruitment or recruitment pattern). This is a neural response to the training stimulus or, put another way, the nerves accommodate to the imposed training loads by firing faster. *Physical changes are absent during this adaptation period.* Only in the presence of *more rigorous stress* will the body be forced to set into motion the process known as muscular "hypertrophy." This will be manifested as muscular growth. Restated, after the efficiency of the nervous system has been optimized, **muscle tissue has no other choice but to grow!**

For all the women out there thinking, "But I don't want to look like a muscle man," let me make an important point. What is the optimal way to **lose body fat** and improve your physique? Aerobics? (you know I despise the word) No. Resistance training. Weight lifting. Female readers are thinking, "But I don't want to bulk up." Ladies, hear me out. You do *not* have the hormonal support to pile on a significant amount of muscle mass. But you will assume a more shapely, much-desired figure should you opt to weight train. You will not be transformed into a bodybuilder. In fact 99.99 percent of men above the age of 30 do NOT have the natural hormonal support to do so either. Please keep in mind that 100 percent of elite professional bodybuilders are on androgenic agents (yes, "steroids" fall into that category). And this is despite their claims of being "natural."

For all you chronic dieters out there, the right strength training program can boost your metabolism and help burn off more fat. By adding muscle to your body, by increasing lean muscle mass, you **increase your basal metabolic rate (BMR)**. It's like taking an additional thermogenic pill. Activated, contracting muscles are the body's furnaces. What is the body's reflexive response to cold exposure? Think. Shivering. And where is the heat generated? In the muscles. Yes the muscle contractions specifically are exothermic processes

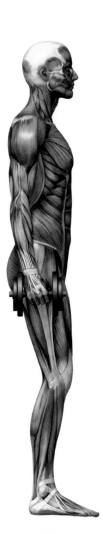

(they release heat) akin to your car heating up as fuel burns within the cylinders. But even at *rest*, your muscle is burning fuel, preferentially fat, in order to maintain itself. And muscle recovering from an intense workout? Even more metabolically active. And therein lies yet another benefit of adding muscle to one's body.

For continual growth to occur, however, a continual and progressive stress must be applied to the muscular system. Similarly, the right nutrition and adequate rest must be provided to allow for such growth. You must force it to change in essence. Why? **Homeostasis**. The body will attempt to minimize energy expenditure and maintain a constant state (of being) or internal equilibrium. From an evolutionary standpoint, such "homeostatic" mechanisms proved beneficial. Conserve energy until there is demand (an attacking predator) or an applied stress (either internal or external). Maintain energy balance. Burn neither fat nor build muscle until you absolutely have to. Simply exist. In the face of a constant, unchanging stress (be it internal or external), the body will adapt and establish a new homeostatic set-point. In other words, the body gets used to a challenge and adapts to it. It stagnates, or hits a plateau, a problem long experienced by dieters. And the "cardio" addicts amongst you...

The fact that walking three miles per day becomes progressively easier is a testimony to bodily adaptation. As a result of the increased efficiency of the body and therefore the lesser energy expenditure, the *benefit of such activity becomes fleeting* as time passes. Ever hear of the law of diminishing returns? Case in point. Applying this dictum to muscular physiology, **only when a progressive (varying) overload is imposed upon the musculoskeletal system, will change occur.**

A Word about Walking

"Well I was told that walking every day does the same thing." No, no, and no. Walking provides little if any metabolic benefit after the fact, as there is no resultant muscular hypertrophy (and relatively little growth factor release).The cardiovascular system will however be stressed, and there is caloric expenditure *while* walking, but less than you may believe. This is why some individuals have difficulty losing weight even while dieting if they simply walk as opposed to weight train (that being said, caution must be exercised when weight training while dieting). Year after year, I watch the same people walk around my neighborhood at 6:30 AM. And year after year, they look no better. Someone famous once said, "Insanity is doing the same thing over and over again but expecting different results."

Nevertheless, I applaud these young ladies' efforts as they are persistent. And consistency is the key. **Health is a lifelong endeavor.** There are no *races* to wellness. On a similar note, you should steer clear of "race-style" fitness regimens. These are fads. You will reap little if any benefit and likely get injured. **Health is a lifestyle.** Only through persistent efforts will you attain your goals. The benefits will only be conferred on the motivated.

Why Muscle Matters

But let's get back to the basics. Why is building a better body so important? What roles does muscle serve? As I will explain, the strength of your musculoskeletal system impacts every aspect of your health.

For one thing, muscle serves a *structural* role. It helps support our skeletal system, our bones and joints. Muscles are attached to their bony points of origin and insertion via tendons. Tendons are comprised of collagen-based connective tissue and are responsive to mechanical stresses, as are ligaments. Ligaments span bony structures and maintain the integrity of the joint structures. For example, an integral ligament of the knee is the anterior cruciate ligament (ACL). The ACL spans the joint space and has origin and insertion points on the femur and tibia, respectively. It controls stability and prevents anterior (forward) movement of the femur relative to the tibia. Such supporting ligaments and the muscles that span a particular joint synergistically function to maintain the integrity of that *particular* joint. Strengthening exercises serve to minimize the stresses placed on the ligaments and reduce the incidence of potentially painful knee injuries. It is also interesting to note that, contrary to popular opinion, physical activity *does not* accelerate degeneration of articular cartilage and may in fact assume rehabilitative (reducing pain in those patients with osteoarthritis) and preventive (preserving joint range of motion) roles. Hence, physical activity is not a predisposition to joint injury. Quite the opposite is true in fact.

No More Bent Over Old Ladies (and Men!)

Strength training is great for your bones too, and that means fewer breaks and fractures. Some 44 million Americans have low bone

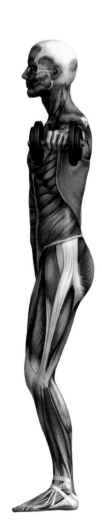

density or osteoporosis, according to the National Osteoporosis Foundation. As a result of this degenerative condition which results in weak and frail bones, about *half* of all women and *one quarter* of men over the age of 50 will break a bone. In rare cases, osteoporosis may be caused by or associated with other diseases and in these cases, it may be inevitable. For the most part, however, the disease is largely preventable. Bone density may be augmented through proper diet and supplementation, the avoidance of certain medications (i.e. warfarin and antacids), and resistance training. Yes, in order to prevent fractures (which can lead to very serious complications, and at times, be fatal) you must train with weights. The spinal column, just like a muscle, becomes stronger in response to your carrying or shouldering a heavy load. Stimulus. Adapative response. Remember? In addition, as even non-postural muscles contract, they exert forces on the bone through tendons. As one's strength and muscle mass increases in response to resistance training, so too must bone mineral density. This is precisely why resistance-trained athletes have higher bone mineral density than age-matched sedentary control subjects. **So start now.** Stop the development of this *preventable* disease in its tracks. It shouldn't require a hip or spine fracture to bring this disease out from under the radar, where it often flies unbeknownst to your personal physician.

Stronger Backs, Fewer Injuries, Less Disease

Want to prevent back injuries? Start strength training. A good strength training program can also **reduce the incidence of low-back injuries,** the most common cause of workplace disability. In addition to the improved quality of life (by remaining injury-free), this translates to a substantial reduction in lost wages and personal medical costs.

By the way, here's an interesting scientific tidbit. The anti-inflammatory effect of exercise (or an applied stress) is paralleled in nature. In late 2008, the

There are a myriad of studies documenting the fact that low-back pain is also reduced with a proper strength training regimen. Interestingly, one study showed a reduction of C-reactive protein (a sensitive blood maker of inflammation) in patients with low-back pain who underwent a multi-component exercise program (which incorporated resistance-training). In addition, participants' back strength and flexibility improved as did leg strength. This study documents the global bodily **anti-inflammatory effect** of a properly employed exercise program and its functional correlate. OK! I hear you! Enough of the doctor talk! ! Simply put, **"YOU FEEL BETTER IF YOU EXERCISE."**

National Science Foundation discovered that walnut trees produce significant amounts of an aspirin-like substance in response to stress. It is postulated that this response helps the plant resist and recover from disease. Get the picture? **Exercise bolsters your resistance to disease.**

Strength Training Is Essential in Physical Therapy

I hope that by staying strong, you avoid most injury, but if you have an existing injury that requires physical therapy, I urge you to make sure that strength training is part of your program. The role of strength training as a **rehabilitative modality** cannot be understated. Unfortunately, the current healthcare system does not consider it as a necessity in both rehabilitative and preventive capacities and reimburses (albeit on a limited basis) for "physical therapy." Sadly, the vast majority of physical therapists have little formal strength training education. Passive range of motion "exercise" is substituted for strength training. And often there is no transition to a strength training regimen. No stress. No adaptation. Poor results. An all too common scenario.

The incorporation of strength training into a rehabilitative program is therefore crucial. Strength training promotes **neuromuscular integrity** (with secondary metabolic gains) and increases joint stability. In the elderly population (often erroneously dissuaded from weight training), this translates into reduced fall risk and a decrease in long bone fractures (Note: There is **NO** documented increased risk of injury in the elderly population who partake in strength training. This is a myth, a fallacy and a farce. In fact, quite the *opposite is true:* injury potential is reduced by a properly applied strength training program). Existing injuries improve. The body's adaptive response is triggered, its capability to heal itself harnessed, at any age.

Get Stronger, Up Your Game

Accordingly, strength training is an integral part of a professional athlete's training regimen, discipline or sport aside. **Every** sport requires strength, physical and mental. Take golf, for example. Undoubtedly more of a mental than physical challenge. But does it surprise you that Tiger Woods places heavy emphasis on strength training? It shouldn't. He is who he is, the elitist amongst the elite because of Lombardian discipline, lifelong practice, a favorable genetic phenotype and the application of sound strength training. Paralleling his ascension to golf's pinnacle, is his noteworthy change in body habitus. Once an ectomorph in every sense of the word, Tiger Woods is now an equally strong physical creature as he is mentally. And likely, his mental game has also improved as a result of the stresses imposed by strength training.

And while it is true that training is "sport-specific" (to be a better golfer, one must practice the sport of *golf*), **proper strength training confers power, speed and endurance** to *all* athletes regardless of their chosen discipline. Baseball players will generate higher bat speeds translating to greater hitting distances. Take, for example, Mark McGuire. Laden with banned substances and sporting an additional 30+ pounds of muscle, he crushed the home run record in 1998, only to be out-done by Barry Bonds (too using anabolic agents) three years later. I am not condoning the use of illegal drugs, however, truth-be-told, strength (and likely bat speed) improvements *afforded* this player the capacity to hit farther. Make no mistake, this was *not* a function of improved batting techniques but purely a factor of power. Strength confers power. Marion Jones, Olympiad, is another case in point.

The development of strength confers an obvious advantage to athletes *regardless of discipline*. A sound strength training regimen should be an adjunct to *every* athlete's training regimen for this reason. Much more worthwhile than ergogenic pills (purchased at health food stores), which promise the world and deliver little, is time spent training, piling on lean muscle, harnessing the adaptive response, and ever-bettering one's self.

But there is no easy way. No pill. It takes hard work. Blood, sweat and tears.
And you will reap the many benefits.

Protects Against Diabetes

A properly executed resistance training program confers protection against disease. This is irrefutable. Resistance training improves glucose tolerance, making one less apt to develop type II diabetes. Its effect on insulin sensitivity is likely multifactorial in etiology but undoubtedly related to the associated increase in lean body mass (through fat loss). That is not to say that thin individuals cannot develop diabetes (and other associated diseases). They can and do. However, 80 percent of individuals with type II diabetes are obese (Obesity is *the* major risk for the development of type II diabetes). And the associated **inflammation** is the underpinning of the vast majority of diseases. I earn a living by treating patients with inflammatory diseases, right? Degenerative spine disease and cancer. Inflammatory in nature. And yes, both diseases are associated with obesity. What is promising however is that obesity can be treated. It, like type II diabetes, is for the most part preventable. Yes there are genetic predispositions to both obesity and the often resultant type II diabetes, *but for the most part*, the ball is in your court. Take the ball and run with it (literally). Stop making excuses as pictured in the above internet circulation.

And while I am not an advocate of running *per se*, short distance sprints are an excellent adjunct to one's resistance training regimen. If performed at proper intervals (no pun intended), such intense bursts of exercise develop strength and power, while concomitantly optimizing the metabolic machinery that removes glucose from our bloodstream. As you'll come to learn, the latter is one of the most important effects of exercise from a health and longevity standpoint.

Enhanced glucose utilization as a direct result of strength training retards the "artery-clogging" or better stated, aging process. Strict glucose control limits the formation of advanced glycation end-products or AGE's, glucose-bound proteins which serve as catalysts for the atherogenic process. By improving insulin sensitivity, resistance training dampens blood sugar spikes and thereby reduces the post-prandial formation of free radicals via a process known as oxidation.

You may be thinking, "I've heard of those "radical" things. They have something to do with aging, yes?"

Stay Younger

Yes. There are a variety of reasons that we as humans age, one of which is oxidant stress from free radical formation. Known as the Free Radical Theory of Aging, this explanation was first proposed by Denham Harman in the 1950s. Other theories include unchecked inflammation, glycation, cell membrane and DNA damage. Interestingly, they are interrelated as I will explain.

Every cell in our body requires energy for a variety of processes. The production of such cellular energy or ATP (adenosine triphosphate) is occurring at the molecular level, unbeknownst to you, billions of times per second, in cellular structures known as mitochondria. Through a complex series of chemical reactions, electrons are ultimately transferred to oxygen, driving the formation of ATP molecules. No oxygen, no electron receptor, death ensues. (Note: Cyanide poisons this so-called "electron transport chain" often times resulting in death.)

This process of ATP generation is imperfect. No one is perfect, right? Well this translates to the molecular level as well. You see, electrons "leak" from the chain prematurely and "reduce" or add electrons to oxygen, ultimately forming free radicals such as the "superoxide anion." The names are unimportant (unless you are a chemist or biophysicist). Understand, however, that free radicals are extremely reactive with their surroundings. Not *inter*active as people are at a town hall meeting, but *re*active. Free radicals react with surrounding molecules like chemicals in a test tube. And unfortunately, the free radicals are the victors. As a super magnet would tear an iron object from one's clutches, so too does a superoxide (or peroxynitrite) radical rob an electron from a molecule of a vital cellular structure. These may be the mitochondrial or cellular membranes which serve a multitude of purposes, let alone a barrier function, or various other cellular organelles, all of which contribute to the inner workings of the cell itself. Free radicals literally "punch holes" in structures through this electrical thievery known as oxidation (loss of an electron). Sounds bad, right? Frenzied molecules piercing adjacent structures and compromising their integrity and potentially their function. Not so fast. We *need* free radicals. Yes, free radicals such as hydrogen peroxide facilitate the elimination of bacterial pathogens that are consumed by our white blood cells. We bleach the suckers to death in essence.

Here's the problem. Free radicals, if produced unchecked, can and do "rust" the body's insides. Oxidation is, after all, the rusting process. We too will rust (or **age**) if our antioxidant systems falter or are overloaded. Remember, the body is smart; it has built-in, highly-effective systems that quench free radicals. We would self-destruct otherwise in their absence, free radicals roaming and scavenging unrestrained. That you are reading this is testimony to the fact that your catalase and superoxide dismutase enzymes are doing a fine job donating electrons to free radicals, satiating the beasts, in lieu of their destroying precious bodily tissue.

Unfortunately, our bodies are exposed to a variety of stimuli, often by choice (or *poor* choice) that promote the formation of excess free radicals. Sugar is a big one as will be discussed in later chapters. Consumption of refined sugars not only fosters the genesis of free radicals but also fuels the fire of inflammation. **And chronic exposure to excess free radicals (oxidation) and inflammation causes age-related disease, period.** Coronary artery disease, the number one killer of Americans? Inflammatory disease. Cancers (those not associated with a particular familial syndrome)? An inflammatory disease characterized by a "runaway" cell line due to DNA damage (from a toxin, UV radiation or free radical). Alzheimer's disease? It has been demonstrated that the brains of Alzheimer's patients are "inflamed." And the list goes on and on. *All diseases have an inflammatory component.* Oxidation and inflammation are like two peas in a pod. Where there's one, there's the other.

   "We have met the enemy and he is us." Barring a massive exposure to radiation, the human body does not assume large quantities of free radicals (also known as reactive oxygen species or ROS) in a single burst. Additionally, as stated above, we possess fairly robust antioxidant systems to maintain our free radical load in check. How do you think George Burns lived to a ripe old age of 100 and smoked incessantly? *Clearly*, he had a free radical scavenging system known only to superheroes and those immune to x-rays, bullets and other environmental insults. Don't bet your life on the off chance that you share George Burns's lucky genetic makeup. Cigarette smoke is laden with free radicals and the majority of us suffer DNA damage (and develop cancer) upon even the smallest exposure to this man-made toxin. Statistically you do not possess the ROS-quenching capacity of George Burns (which was likely due to a protective overexpression of his antioxidant enzymes) and therefore could use some assistance in your quest to live to 100. Strength training to the rescue. Again. Yet another benefit of strength training is an augmented antioxidant capacity. (But you still shouldn't smoke... ever.)

   We don't want these reactive oxygen species running rampant, right? Well, then you've got to run them off. Sprint. Short-interval sprints. Intense, burst-type running and strength training bolsters one's antioxidant systems. This was recently demonstrated in a 2012 study that assayed enzymatic activity and quantified oxidative stress in response to a progressive resistance training regimen. Superoxide dismutase activity, a deficiency of which has been implicated in the genesis of Lou Gehrig's Disease (ALS), was significantly increased in the red blood cells of those individuals who trained for eight weeks. And this phenomenon has been *repeatedly* demonstrated. *Exercise strengthens our defense systems, plain and simple.*

   This should come as no surprise to you either. Individuals who exercise are exposed to the associated oxidative stresses and *adapt to those stresses* by up-regulating antioxidant enzymes. Stress and adaptive response. This confers protection against the free radical onslaught that accompanies muscle contraction. But this effect is not limited to the muscles. There are fringe benefits. *Total body* antioxidant capacity is augmented. This is manifested as **disease regression** and externally as tighter skin (as it is less susceptible to free radical damage).

But Don't "Stress-Out"

That being said, we've all witnessed those individuals in our "more is better" society who insist on doing ultra-marathons or running long distances, chronically. Most appear worn and lacking in muscle mass. They look older than their chronological years. Because they are! They have accelerated the aging process dramatically by exposing their bodies to excessive free radical loads associated with these 100-mile jaunts. The endogenous antioxidant systems are simply overloaded and can't keep up! While I understand the draw of such endurance challenges, the big picture must be kept in mind. This is about health after all. And while you may gravitate towards such events based upon your predominant muscle fiber-type (i.e. type I), skip it. Your body will thank you for it in the long run (no pun intended).

I would strongly recommend that you utilize your time strength training instead. This will grant you the shape you desire (and not the skeletal-wasted look of the aged runner) and concomitantly optimize your hormones, many of which decline with age. Chronic endurance training, in addition to burdening your body with heavy free radical loads, also has deleterious effects on your hormones, cortisol for example. This stress hormone is produced in the adrenal gland and is secreted in response to exercise of any type. While cortisol is to a great degree responsible for our flight or fight response, excessively high levels on a chronic basis can predispose us to "overtraining" and ultimately adrenal (neuroendocrine) fatigue, compromising our immune system and predisposing us to disease. Abuse of our cortisol-based *defense* system therefore yields quite the opposite effect, making us more susceptible to illness and injury. And while the overtraining syndrome affects mainly endurance athletes, it too may develop in response to an aggressive resistance training program. For a variety of reasons, this being one of them, I purposely limit endurance work in my training regimen (as to not induce excessive bodily stress). Remember one of the goals of a training program is to restore a youthful hormone profile. Often times, endurance training is guilty of just the opposite.

Default to resistance training as *the* primary modality therefore. [Use endurance training *only* as an adjunct to maintain a reasonable level of cardiovascular fitness. Everyone should be capable of running a mile and a half without much difficulty, *regardless* of muscle mass. (I've always used this benchmark as a poor man's stress test.)] Resistance training, specifically the induced muscular trauma, stimulates the release of reparative hormones such as testosterone and growth hormone. Present in both males and females, these hormones appear to augment the individual's ability to tolerate and sustain prolonged high exercise intensities, in essence better preparing him for the next battle. Unfortunately, levels of these hormones decline with age. Or do we age as a result of their decline? I prefer to assume the latter in this "chicken and egg" debate, having personally observed the restorative effects of hormone replacement therapy (HRT). Face it, the re-establishment of youthful hormonal balance is associated with a reduction in body fat, increased muscle mass, heightened energy and libido, and improved sleep habits. Who wouldn't want that? No one...

By driving the synthesis and release of growth hormone, testosterone and DHEA, resistance training exerts effects similar to exogenous hormone replacement, albeit on a smaller scale. Accordingly, the best way to increase your testosterone naturally is to well... lift weights! The heightened levels of these hormones will increase muscle mass and serve to reduce body fat. This is of utmost importance in the aged population in whom resistance training has been demonstrated to attenuate muscle wasting and improve resistance to debility. In the context of that said earlier, endurance training, which is the best exercise to increase/maintain mitochondrial concentration with aging, has generally resulted in relatively small *functional* benefits to nursing home patients. I'd rather see YOU, the healthy 95-year-old, performing 50 body weight squats daily than walking a mile.

Compound (multi-joint), weight-bearing exercises such as the squat, dramatically improve body composition due to the significant demands placed on the body. In the presence of adequate nutrition, muscle will hypertrophy, and by virtue, total body protein stores will increase. This results in improved healing capacity and augmented immunity. One's immune system relies upon body protein stores to form antibodies; *muscle in essence acts as a fuel source for the immune system.* In this context, numerous studies have demonstrated the importance of muscle mass in the survival of critically ill patients. Additionally, a landmark study in the *British Medical Journal* published in 2008 demonstrated that *muscular strength is inversely and independently associated with death from **all causes and cancer** in men,* even after adjusting for cardiorespiratory fitness and other potential confounders.

The profound impact that strength training has on all-cause mortality and cancer is likely multifactorial in origin. Strength training, as stated earlier, has very profound anti-inflammatory effects. While the recovery from an intense workout is dependent on one's ability to mount an *inflammatory* response, this tissue repair process is short-term, a by-product of **acute** inflammation. These transient periods of inflammation are attenuated by the production of anti-inflammatory cytokines (immune system signaling molecules), thereby facilitating muscle recovery. Of course, ample time must be allotted between bouts of heavy exercise in order to *allow* for recovery to occur, or else over-training, a syndrome of **chronic** inflammation, may occur. This is akin to an accelerated aging process given the heightened bodily inflammation and persistently elevated serum cortisol levels. Avoid it at all costs!

Similarly, resistance training improves the body's ability to control free radicals. Remember those nasty free radicals (ROS) released during exercise? Often the bad guys, ROS also serve as signal molecules which up-regulate the body's antioxidant capacity, as does lactate (lactic acid) generated during resistance training.

That burn you feel during exercise, particularly strength-endurance work? Celebrate it. **Chase it down!** Intense exercise such as sprint-intervals exerts protective effects on the cardiovascular system. A healthy cardiovascular system translates to improved longevity and lesser disease burden. Remember "you are only as old as your arteries."

Exercise Boosts Brain Power

This applies to the brain as well as the heart. Stroke and vascular dementia are associated with significant worldwide morbidity and mortality. As discussed earlier, risk factors for cerebrovascular disease are *no different* than those for cardiovascular disease. Surprise, surprise! And most of the risk factors are modifiable: high blood pressure, cigarette smoking, diabetes mellitus, dyslipidemia, poor nutrition and physical inactivity/obesity. An optimal diet and daily exercise can temper free radical load and quell inflammation and glycation. And while there are genetic predispositions to diseases such as Alzheimer's dementia, **you** can still mitigate your risk through these two modalities, as discussed throughout this book.

Exercise has been demonstrated to alter the progression of Alzheimer's and Parkinson's disease. These beneficial effects are thought to be related to an augmented antioxidant status, increased cerebral blood flow, and potentially enhanced neurogenesis. Yes, you have the capacity to form new neurons and synapses (neuronal interconnections) throughout your life if you remain active physically! And by virtue of this, by mitigating the effects of neuronal loss, exercise plays a preventive role against neurodegenerative diseases.

Therefore, at the cellular level, exercise "works" the brain. Synapses are formed and connections to the peripheral nervous system are reinforced. By acquiring the skills to execute a perfect deadlift or squat, you forge neural pathways through the corticospinal pathway which links brain to muscle. These connections are reinforced through training and manifested as bettered performance (and often times, a more stalwart physique). Leaner, stronger and mentally sharper you will be. Your focus will intensify in parallel to the rigors of training. And this will translate to tasks outside the gym. You will exhibit a renewed sense of well-being and confidence. Could you otherwise attempt that heavy bench press? Lacking self-confidence, no. You must **know** that you will succeed **prior** to lying down on the bench, as integral to physical strength is mental strength. **An iron body begins with an iron mind.**

Fulfillment of your fitness dreams (whatever they may be) will come with time, patience and persistence. Your brain is "plastic" even during your later years. You have within you the capability of altering your brain which will secondarily alter your body, *at any age*. Remember what triggers your muscles to lift that heavy weight. It's resident between your ears! Yet it doesn't know how to hoist that heavy barbell off the ground until you teach it, until you acquire that skill. This learning process occurs over a *lifetime*. Strength. Health. *Lifetime* endeavors. Most people don't appreciate this, however, and cancel their gym memberships for lack of *immediate* results. That's akin to quitting health.

Stick with it instead.

Be willing to do what others won't.

Claim your health.

Get Serious!

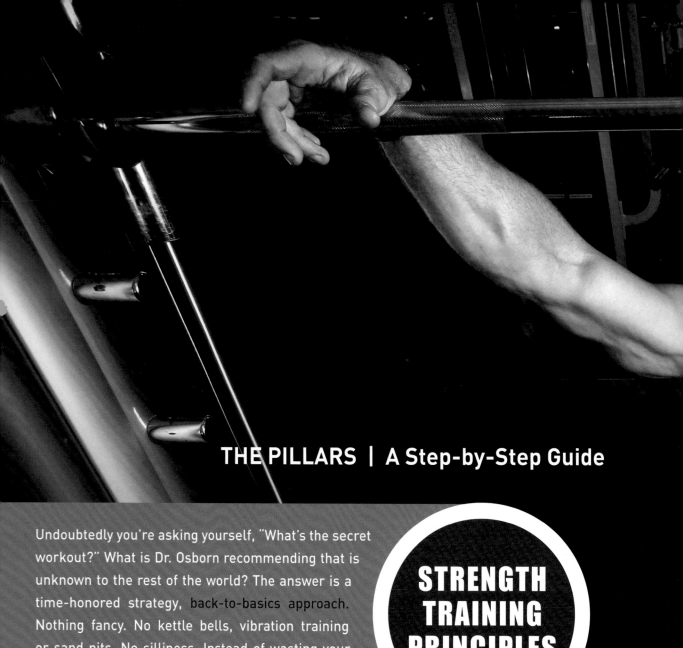

THE PILLARS | A Step-by-Step Guide

Undoubtedly you're asking yourself, "What's the secret workout?" What is Dr. Osborn recommending that is unknown to the rest of the world? The answer is a time-honored strategy, back-to-basics approach. Nothing fancy. No kettle bells, vibration training or sand pits. No silliness. Instead of wasting your time with the "latest and greatest" fitness program, consider developing a sound knowledge base *first*.

STRENGTH TRAINING PRINCIPLES

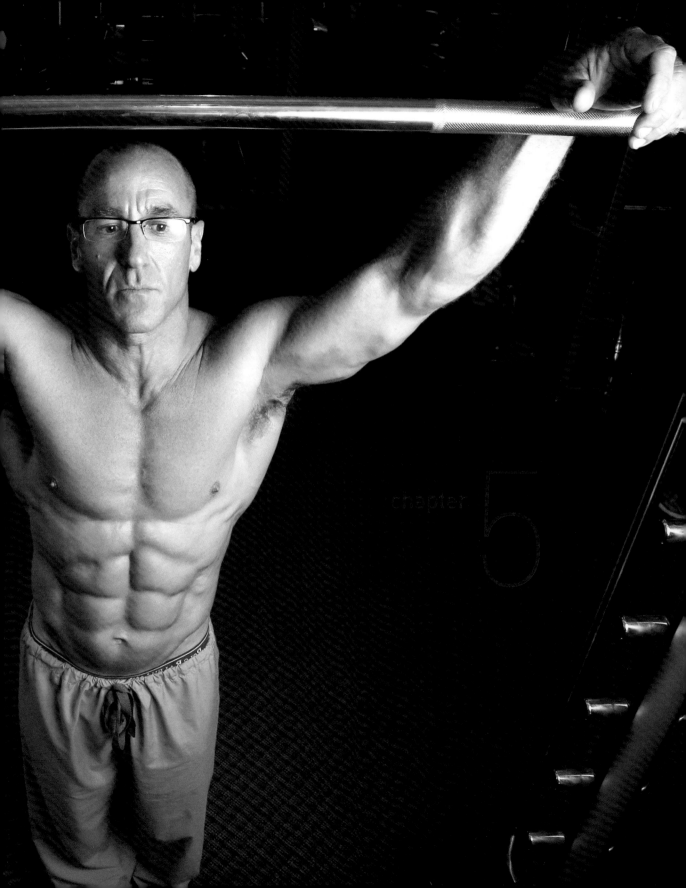

I am here to help you help yourself. I will tell you *why* I have chosen these specific exercises. My goal is not to sell you the merits of the exercises but to show you how and why a "foundational" approach through basic movements is *always* best. I recommend a few basic movements that engage the biggest muscle groups in the most effective, efficient way. Sure, certain movements may be utilized as adjuncts, but the pillars of the training regimen will always be the five basic compound movements: **squat, bench press, deadlift, overhead press and a chin/pull-up or rowing movement.**

Intimate knowledge of these exercises is a must. You must understand which muscles are activated, the mechanics of the movement itself, proper execution, and pitfalls. First and foremost, however, is injury prevention and their management should they occur. Remember, it's **injury prevention first, get strong second.** An injury can set you back months. Take it from me, I've been there.

The five foundational exercises target the larger muscle groups of the body, and by virtue of this generate a significant anabolic response (hormonal). The more muscle traumatized (electively) during a training session, the greater the hormonal (adaptive or reparative) response. For example, I think wrist curls, which engage only a few isolated muscles, are a waste of time, even if performed at the highest intensity. On the other hand, a set of deep squats, which engage nearly every muscle group in the body, is more beneficial even if performed at a low to moderate intensity. So scrap the wrist curls. Seek out those movements that provide the biggest bang for the buck: squats, deadlifts, overhead press, bench press and chin/pull-ups or a rowing movement. Whatever your goals: if you want to be big and muscular, or if you want to be nicely toned and sculpted, these basic exercises will get the job done. No balls or bikes or bands needed. Nothing fancy. It's easier than you think, although it does take work and dedication. But what else is more important than your health? **NOTHING!** After all, it's why you're reading this book, right?

So, let's begin.

Several critical points must be emphasized initially. These will be explained in detail as your understanding of them is mandatory. The majority of individuals who fail to make physical gains are guilty of violating one *or more* of these rules. Yet instead of asking why, they simply quit (go figure!). Therefore, *always* default to the following principles and assure adherence to them prior to further introspection. Likely you'll find the answer right here.

RULE #1 INTENSITY

Training must be intense. Jack LaLanne described exercise as "systematic, vigorous, and violent." More scientifically stated, *any exercise or group of exercises must provide sufficient stimulus to trigger the body's adaptive response.* A requisite of this is "intensity."

We are reactive organisms at base level. The environment (which includes the food we ingest) presents a signal, and we react to the signal. And the process repeats. This "signal processing" is extremely complex and mediated by a myriad of biochemical processes. Our genes provide the precise regulatory instructions. They govern the processes by turning protein synthesis on and off within a particular cell. At base level, we are the products of our genes, and these have remained essentially static for the last 10,000 years. However, whether or not specific proteins are translated (produced within our cells) is a function of the intracellular environment (whether or not the cell is stressed, for example) and the extracellular environment (the environment immediately outside the cell). Food, good or bad, serves to signal the translation of certain proteins (insulin, for example). Hormones such as testosterone also serve as signal molecules by interacting with receptors (within the nucleus) that directly bind genes regulating muscle protein synthesis.

As such, resistance training of sufficient intensity stimulates an increase in testosterone production, and the anabolic (muscle-building) process ensues. Muscle injury at the cellular level is in part responsible for the anabolic signaling that occurs in the post-exercise period. The inflammatory process is invoked as well (after all, resistance training is induced trauma or injury to the muscular structures). One's recovery from a training session is dependent, therefore, on the integrity of the acute (and I stress, *acute*) inflammatory process. Without it, you simply will not recover. Muscular soreness that you may experience 48 hours post-exercise is simply the result of the inflammatory repair process. It's normal. We adapt to the stresses that are imposed upon our bodies. Again, "that which does not kill us makes us stronger."

Productive exercise (uncommonly seen in gyms today) serves to "turn the genetic switch" on. *If you exercise with a lack of intensity, you may as well stay home.* Intense exercise generates a stimulus to which the body responds over the ensuing days to weeks (depending on one's recovery ability). Recovery from the insult is dependent on one's nutritional status, quality sleep, and ample time allotment between workouts. Enter Arthur Jones...

RULE #2 NEUROMUSCULAR STIMULUS

Jones, the founder of Nautilus, Inc. and the inventor of numerous novel pieces of exercise equipment, championed the idea that high intensity exercise performed infrequently would effect maximal strength gains if dosed properly (as per an individual's recovery capacity). Thousands of hours of research allowed him to formulate training protocols based upon this "less is more" philosophy. Again, trigger the adaptive response ("turn the switch on") and allow the body to respond. Do not again train the same body part(s) until recovery is complete, else you will recognize few if any gains.

While I am not an advocate of short-sessions, once or twice weekly full-body Jones-style workouts (except for use on an intermittent basis), I wholeheartedly agree with his philosophy. Specifically, there is a certain minimal quantity of neuromuscular stimulation which will effect gains. One should seek out this level of stimulation (and nothing more) through intense training. Because more is not better. Don't believe the hype! In fact, "more" will only predispose you to overtraining and stalled progress. As such, *always err on the side of training less.*

So how do you know just how much is enough? Are you training too often or just the opposite? In both cases, there will be failed gains. The answer? Experience and meticulous attention to your progress (or lack thereof). In that vein, I give you the next rule.

RULE #3 PROGRESS

Chart your progress.

You don't know where you're going unless you know where you've been. Nothing new here. Yet why is it that the overwhelming majority of people engaged in a weight training regimen do not (nor have not) logged their workouts. Ever hear of goal-directed behavior? There is no progress without record of past accomplishments. This is critical. Buy a log book or download an app (there are many available for free) and make a habit of recording every workout. Don't follow the masses. Most people wander about the gym aimlessly having decided to "do chest" that day. The protocols they use (exercises, weights and rep schemes) are determined on-the-fly (no pun intended), if you will. There is no plan. There is no structure to the workout. And those people look the same (physically) year after year after year. Do you fall into that category? No plan. No progress. Just aimless wandering around the gym. Now take control. *Set training goals* (short-term and long-term) and *accomplish them.* Let nothing stand in your way! This will prove impossible, however, if you ignore the next rule.

RULE #4 NUTRITION

You must provide your body with adequate nutrition to rebuild itself should this be your fitness goal (muscular hypertrophy and strength). In fact, **nutrition is of equal importance to the training stimulus.** You will make few if any gains in the context of poor nutrition. Think about it. Your recovering muscles are demanding protein and yet you serve them Skittles. It doesn't matter that your caloric intake is in excess of your basal metabolic rate (BMR). Yes, you'll gain weight, but I can assure you that the additional weight will be added to your spare tire instead of your biceps! If you want to add muscle, traumatize the muscle appropriately through intense training and provide it with adequate protein to optimize recovery. Don't scratch your head when your performance in the gym stinks. Instead, reassess your diet for the past week. Likely the problem will be staring you in the face. Statistically speaking, it's either nutrition or this next issue which stalls progress.

RULE #5 SLEEP

I'm guilty of this one by virtue of my occupation: inadequate sleep. Part and parcel with sound nutrition is obtaining adequate rest. **You must get adequate sleep.** You simply won't recover otherwise. Remember, you are growing while you sleep (provided there is adequate stimulus for growth and in the context of sound nutrition). Lack of sleep will predispose you to overtraining (if your workout frequency is not appropriately tailored back). This will result in stalled progress, bodily fatigue, and predisposition to illness. And forget about packing on that desired muscle, as lack of sleep has been associated with obesity! Make every effort to obtain eight hours of sound sleep. Your body and mind will thank you for it.

RULE #6 EDUCATE YOURSELF

Learn as much as possible about training and more specifically how your body responds to various training modalities. Don't scour the fitness or fashion magazines in search of the latest and greatest exercise routine. The endorsed regimens in bodybuilding magazines bear little resemblance to those actually utilized by bodybuilders. And unless you are on massive amounts of androgens, you will have significant difficulty recovering from the high-volume work promulgated by these giants. And those "lose 15 pounds in a week" celebrity diet/workout plans are equally unrealistic if not downright dangerous. Ignore shows such as "The Biggest Loser." Understand that the contestants' weight loss is comprised of both fat and muscle, something you want to avoid at all costs (remember, muscle is protective). Their weekly weight losses are extremely aggressive, set unrealistic expectations for the viewers, and teach the contestants little about their individual physiologies (something they should glean from *their* experiences). It's not about generating a caloric deficit through vigorous exercise and therefore catabolizing your entire body, muscle included. That's precisely what you want to avoid! Analyze everything. Understand the pitfalls of these glamorized, often illogical fitness regimens. And if something does not make perfect sense, well... call bullshit and walk away.

RULE #7 NEVER QUIT!

But don't quit. **Never quit!** This is the most important rule. A well-timed hiatus from training is very different than quitting. In fact, we need intermittent breaks as the majority of us, believe it or not, are overtraining. Terminating all exercise is akin to quitting health. You must push yourself through periods of stalled progress. Men, don't expect to look like a professional bodybuilder after 6-12 months of training. It is likely that you will never amass even half of their lean muscle without the use of anabolic agents. And that's OK! Your goal is slow, yet steady progression in the weight room which will translate into a more muscular physique and ultimately bettered health.

And women, you may not fit into your size 2 jeans in two weeks, and maybe not ever. But you will look a lot better and feel great within a few months of regimented training. And you will be much stronger, healthier, and less likely to fall prey to disease. So keep going.

Set short-term training goals and refer often to your workout log. Strength gains will be readily apparent! And these should be motivating enough. Each week, you will lift just a bit heavier and in time, these "paper" gains will equate to physical gains. People will take note! And this will drive you harder. And discourage you from quitting. Ever...

The following photos highlight the finer technical points of the five pillar exercises. Collectively, they should **NOT** serve as a replacement for a skilled trainer. **All of the demonstrated movements should be supervised by and perfected in conjunction with a trainer. The author assumes no responsibility for injuries incurred.** In this context, your priorities should be as follows:

SAFETY FIRST, GET STRONG SECOND

Featured in the photos is Renée Halfhill, LPT, President and CEO of Blue Sky Therapy in Canfield, Ohio. With a passion for rehabilitation and fitness, Renée is in spectacular shape at age 52! She is a true testimony to the fact that women can be sexy *and* strong too. Yes ladies, you can do it, at any age...

And here's another tidbit. I wanted a photo of a *woman* doing a chin-up. Why? Because it is challenging, even for a man. Renée couldn't do one rep. *Six weeks later,* with some coaching and encouragement, she performed four! This is an amazing feat. Now see for yourself. She is truly an inspiration (even to me).

WORKOUT SPECIFICS

The Appendix details a comprehensive training regimen that may be utilized by both novice and advanced trainees. The program logically intertwines resistance and cardiovascular training in order to promote strength gains while accelerating fat loss. I've utilized this program (and variations thereof) for years with nothing short of dramatic results. Now **Get Serious. Get going!**

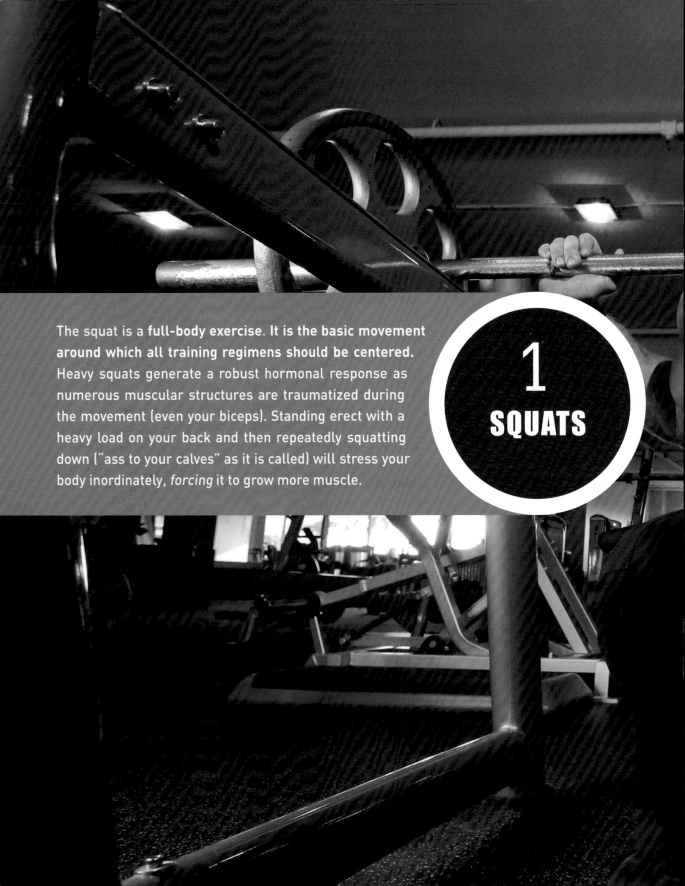

The squat is a **full-body exercise. It is the basic movement around which all training regimens should be centered.** Heavy squats generate a robust hormonal response as numerous muscular structures are traumatized during the movement (even your biceps). Standing erect with a heavy load on your back and then repeatedly squatting down ("ass to your calves" as it is called) will stress your body inordinately, *forcing* it to grow more muscle.

1
SQUATS

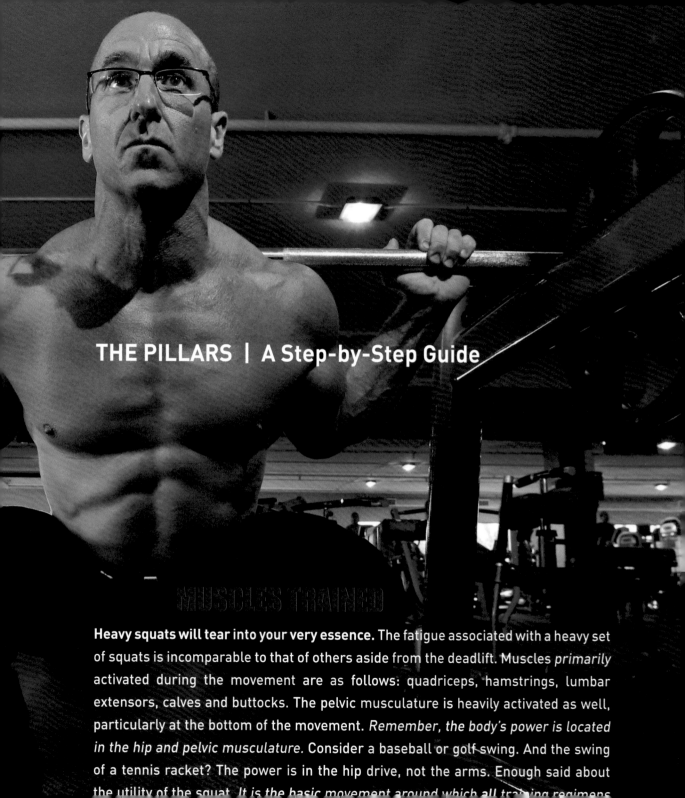

THE PILLARS | A Step-by-Step Guide

MUSCLES TRAINED

Heavy squats will tear into your very essence. The fatigue associated with a heavy set of squats is incomparable to that of others aside from the deadlift. Muscles *primarily* activated during the movement are as follows: quadriceps, hamstrings, lumbar extensors, calves and buttocks. The pelvic musculature is heavily activated as well, particularly at the bottom of the movement. *Remember, the body's power is located in the hip and pelvic musculature.* Consider a baseball or golf swing. And the swing of a tennis racket? The power is in the hip drive, not the arms. Enough said about the utility of the squat. *It is the basic movement around which all training regimens*

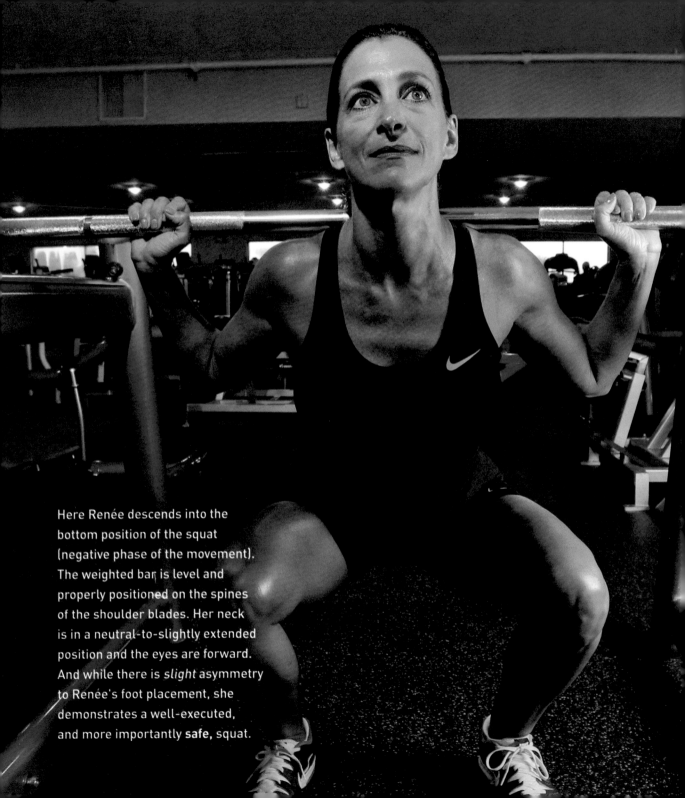

Here Renée descends into the
bottom position of the squat
(negative phase of the movement).
The weighted bar is level and
properly positioned on the spines
of the shoulder blades. Her neck
is in a neutral-to-slightly extended
position and the eyes are forward.
And while there is *slight* asymmetry
to Renée's foot placement, she
demonstrates a well-executed,
and more importantly **safe**, squat.

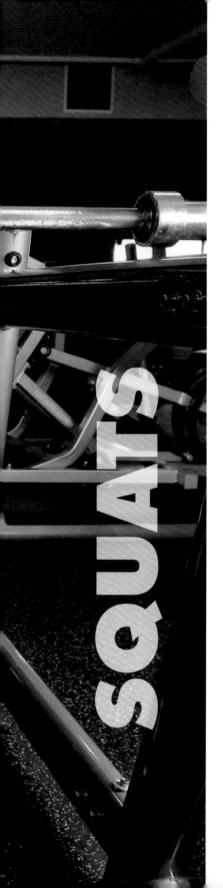

THIS IS UNDOUBTEDLY THE KING OF ALL EXERCISES.

Volumes have been written on the technical aspects of the squat. It stresses the *entire body*. That being said, guys, if you want to add an inch to your *arms*, squat. Women, if you want to have great "no jiggle" sleek arms, squat. You heard me. Squat! Heavy squats generate a robust hormonal response as numerous muscular structures are traumatized during the movement (even your biceps). Standing erect with a heavy load on your back and then repeatedly squatting down, will stress your body inordinately, **forcing it to grow more muscle.** You leave it little room to run in essence. That being said, your training progress will be suboptimal should squats be excluded from your regimen. *So don't even think about it.* And no, you cannot exchange leg extensions for squats. If this was even a consideration, reread the paragraph. And then read it again, as you missed the point. And no, squats if performed properly are not dangerous, nor are they "bad for your back." Take it from someone who has done well over 1,000 spine operations.

SAFETY CONSIDERATIONS

Seek the advice of an experienced squatter. Learn form and proper technique *primarily*. This will translate to safety. Do not even consider loading your back with a weighted bar if you have sustained a recent spine fracture or disc herniation, have been diagnosed with osteoporosis, or have not been cleared by your doctor (for any preclusive medical condition).

Novice squatters should *always* squat with a spotter *and* in a squat rack or cage. More advanced trainees often forego a spotter, although this is not recommended when working with near 1 RM (1-rep maximum) weight loads or during high-rep sets (as fatigue may set in fairly rapidly).

You may *consider* wearing a weight belt particularly if you have injured your low back in the past. This is suggestive of weakened lumbar extensor muscles which will be heavily stressed during a proper squat movement. Applying this logic, I tend to squat without a belt in order to augment my low-back strength (making me less predisposed to future sprain/strain injuries). However, if you are apprehensive about exposing your low back to the inherent stresses of the squat (as the lumbar musculature is *what* keeps you from falling forward during the movement), by all means, use your belt. It will certainly bolster the stability of your mid-section.

Warm-up sets are critical. Work sets are to be preceded by multiple preparatory sets beginning with the unloaded Olympic bar (45 pounds) and escalating in poundage to the target weight. Directly shouldering heavy training loads ("cold") will result in failed squat attempts and predispose you to injury.

EXERCISE TECHNIQUE

As with any exercise, **form is critical.** Squatting is an unnatural movement and potentially places the lumbar spine at risk *if* performed improperly. That being said, it is extremely safe *if* you adhere to proper technique.

1 Focus on the task at hand. See yourself through the movement before even approaching the weighted bar on the squat rack. Assure that your spotter is ready.

EXERCISE TECHNIQUE CONTINUED

2 Approach the racked bar (which should be at armpit height), placing it evenly across the top of the posterior deltoids (and just below the spine of the scapula). The bar should literally lie on top of the bony prominences of your shoulder blades. Reach back and feel them prior to your first squat attempt! Grasp the bar with either a thumbless or closed-handed grip.

3 Position your feet *directly* under the bar slightly wider than shoulder-width apart. You will be in a slight squat at this point, although the lumbar region should be in extension (and *never* rounded).

4 Flare your elbows back to secure the bar in position. The resulting forward pressure (at the hands) will assist you in maintaining the load on your shoulders while concomitantly "unweighting" your arms.

5 To unrack the bar, simply extend the hips and knees. Carefully yet deliberately, bear the loaded bar. You should be standing upright at this point. If you have never shouldered a bar before, it may seem heavy or awkward. *That's normal.* Keep going.

6 Assuming you are not squatting in a cage (but in a rack), you will be required to take several steps backwards prior to beginning the first rep. Be extremely careful doing so even in the context of light bar loads. I have witnessed injuries during this setup phase. For this and a variety of other reasons, squats should be performed in a cage. Nevertheless...

7 After you have reached your final position in the apparatus, feet slightly wider than shoulder-width, externally rotate feet (turn your toes outward) by approximately 30 degrees. You are ready to begin the descent.

8 With an arched back and *weight centered directly over your heels,* flex your hips and knees while maintaining lumbar extension. Inhale just prior to your descent.

9 Better put by Mark Rippetoe, renowned collegiate strength and conditioning coach, "sit back, lean forward and shove your knees out." Yes, lean forward, slightly. Squats are *not* performed with a vertical posture as is often taught. This will simply make the hip drive inefficient.

10 The bottom position of the squat is reached when the top of your thighs is just slightly past parallel (to the floor), *not before.* You will experience a sensation of stretching as the quadriceps, muscles of the "posterior chain," and calves are reaching their range limits. The stored potential energy in these muscles (in the form of a stretch reflex) assists in the so-called "hip drive."

11 Without changing your posture, raise your butt straight up, neither forward nor backward, but *straight up.* This will initiate the positive (concentric) phase of the movement.

12 Now drive the bar to the finish position, maintaining a rigid posture and your weight over the mid-foot. It is simply a matter of "standing up" properly by extending the hips and knees. The bar should be driven out of the bottom in a vertical line. This will allow for maximal power transfer (and little wasted energy).

13 Exhale. The Valsalva maneuver (forceful attempted expiration against a closed airway which is similar but not identical to a "breath hold") is employed transiently *during* the lift in order to stabilize the lumbar spine, thereby providing better energy transfer from body to bar. You won't die of an "aneurysm" as is commonly portrayed. Take it from a neurosurgeon.

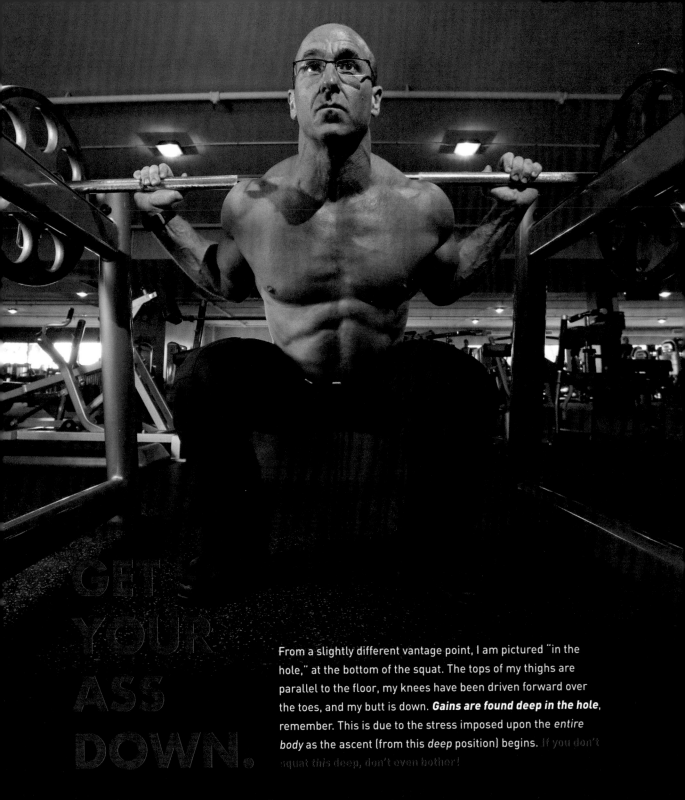

GET YOUR ASS DOWN.

From a slightly different vantage point, I am pictured "in the hole," at the bottom of the squat. The tops of my thighs are parallel to the floor, my knees have been driven forward over the toes, and my butt is down. *Gains are found deep in the hole*, remember. This is due to the stress imposed upon the *entire body* as the ascent (from this *deep* position) begins. If you don't squat *this deep*, don't even bother!

PITFALLS

Allowing your center of mass to come forward onto your toes. This is a big one. Are your heels off the ground during the descent? The solution is *not* squatting with a block under your heels as trainees are often instructed. The solution is: fix the problem.

Learn to "sit into the squat" even if you are tall. Your knees should track out over your toes, no farther, while your buttocks descend into the so-called "hole." You'll experience a sinking sensation. That is your trigger to begin the ascent, as your femur has just passed the plane parallel to the floor. The drive out of the bottom of the squat is initiated with vertical hip drive, lifting you out of the "hole," ass-first.

A "knock-kneed" ascent out of the bottom. Obviously, this problem results in impaired power transfer from body to bar. You simply are wasting energy driving the knees together as opposed to extending them during the ascent. Easily fixed.

Assure that your feet are externally rotated as above. This will facilitate knee tracking over the feet. Additionally, attempt to "externally rotate" your thighs during your descent. This will be impossible as your feet are firmly planted on the ground but will nevertheless drive your knees outward.

Allowing hyperflexion of the lumbar spine. Dangerous. And 100 percent preventable. I've seen people slammed to the floor having fallen forward during both phases of the squat. Why? *Several reasons:*
1. Weak lumbar extensor muscles
2. Rapid hip drive out of the bottom (in a backwards direction) with asynchronous hip and knee extension.

The descent (eccentric or negative phase of the movement) is of equal or greater importance than the drive (concentric phase) of the squat. It is the setup for the drive and therefore must be technically sound. *During the descent (as well as the ascent), the alignment of the lumbar spine does not change. Specifically, neutral alignment is maintained.* What is neutral lumbar alignment? Lordosis (the medical term for an inward curvature of the spine) or extension. Take a look at a model of the spine. Specifically note the lumbar anatomy. Do you see how the lumbar spine appears as to be "leaning back" in mild extension? Not hyperextension and certainly not flexion. To maintain this alignment during the squat, one must possess a certain degree of lumbar extensor strength which prevents the shoulders from slumping forward. This averts potentially exposing the lifter to the dangers of round-back lifting. Remember, most lumbar injuries outside the gym environment occur as a result of round-back lifting (often times at awkward angles). So how is lumbar extensor strength developed? Hmm... Squatting.

The lumbar musculature will be similarly (and unnecessarily) stressed if the hips are driven backwards instead of vertically during the initial part of the ascent, particularly if the hip and knee extension lag and are unable to right the weight. The low back will rapidly assume a more horizontal, flexed position, diminishing (or eliminating) power transfer from legs to bar and predisposing you to injury. Don't do this! *Ass goes straight up out the bottom, period.*

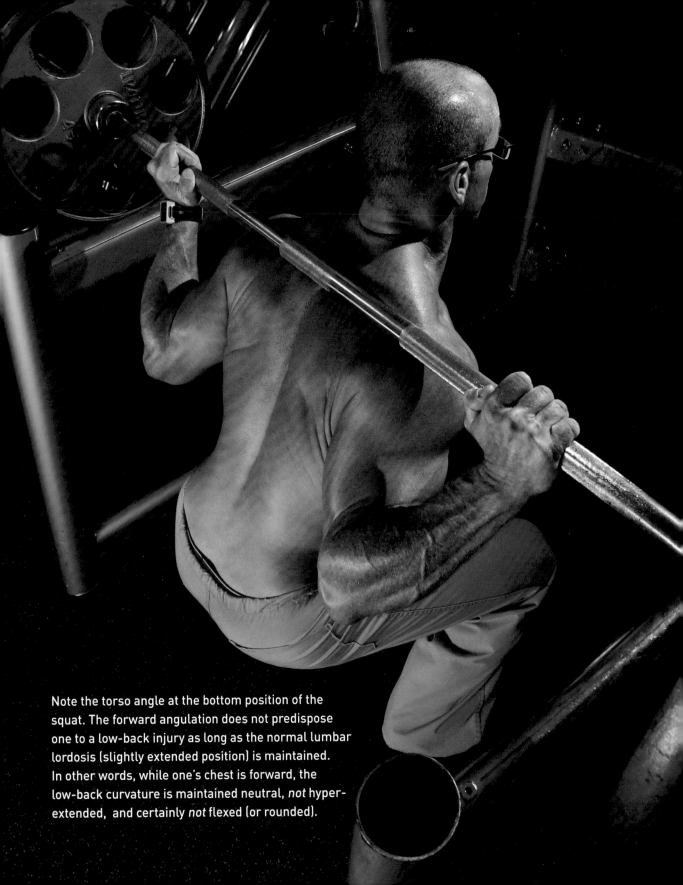

Note the torso angle at the bottom position of the squat. The forward angulation does not predispose one to a low-back injury as long as the normal lumbar lordosis (slightly extended position) is maintained. In other words, while one's chest is forward, the low-back curvature is maintained neutral, *not* hyper-extended, and certainly *not* flexed (or rounded).

SQUATTING REQUIRES PRACTICE. It is a technical lift which, if mastered, will *dramatically* affect your training results. Squatting is not to be neglected (but emphasized in fact) if you are physically capable! Expend extra effort learning the nuances of the movement from an expert. Strive for perfect form, as this will confer safety and allow for continued progress. And remember, there are no shortcuts: partial squats with 405 lbs. are far less beneficial than are deep squats with 315 lbs. Beginners, I'd rather see you squat deep with an unloaded bar than do a half squat with 95 lbs. The money is at the bottom, deep in the hole. There gains sleep. **So Get Serious and get squatting...**

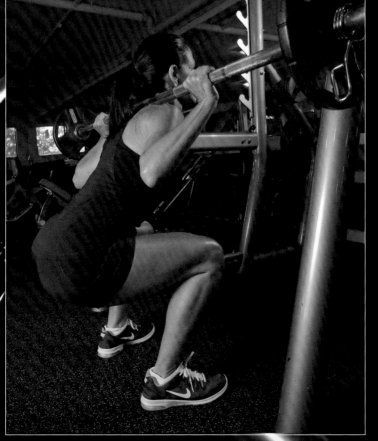

The forward angulation of the torso (and the low position of the bar on the spines of the scapulae) allows the bar to ascend and descend in a straight vertical path, maximizing efficiency and power transfer from the ground to the bar. Your lumbar musculature (extensors) will be strengthened by *maintaining* this position during the squat. This will in turn minimize your chances of a low-back injury. So ignore what you've been told about squats! **Properly performed, there is no better exercise. End of Discussion.**

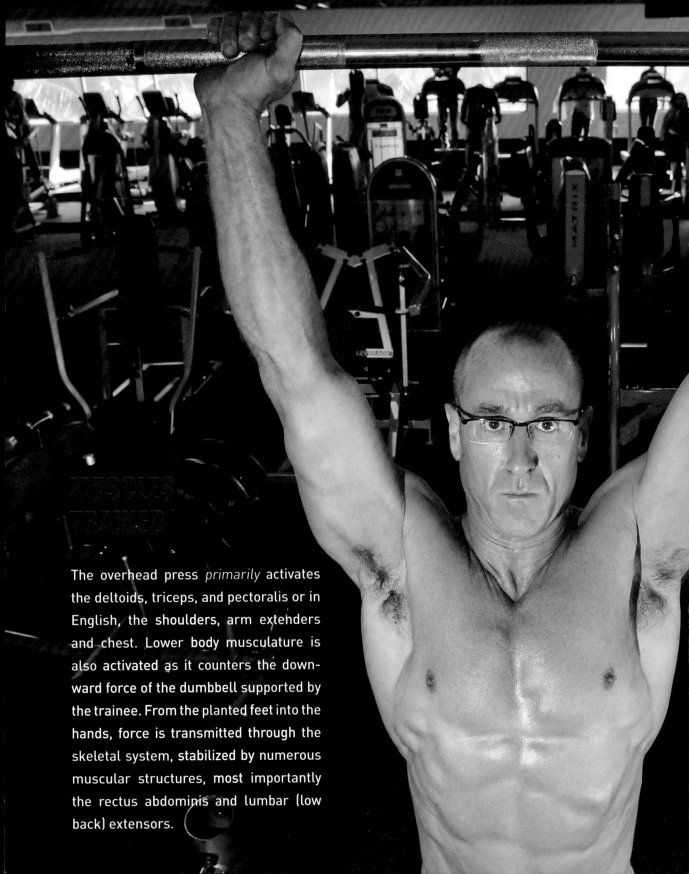

The overhead press *primarily* activates the deltoids, triceps, and pectoralis or in English, the shoulders, arm extenders and chest. Lower body musculature is also activated as it counters the downward force of the dumbbell supported by the trainee. From the planted feet into the hands, force is transmitted through the skeletal system, stabilized by numerous muscular structures, most importantly the rectus abdominis and lumbar (low back) extensors.

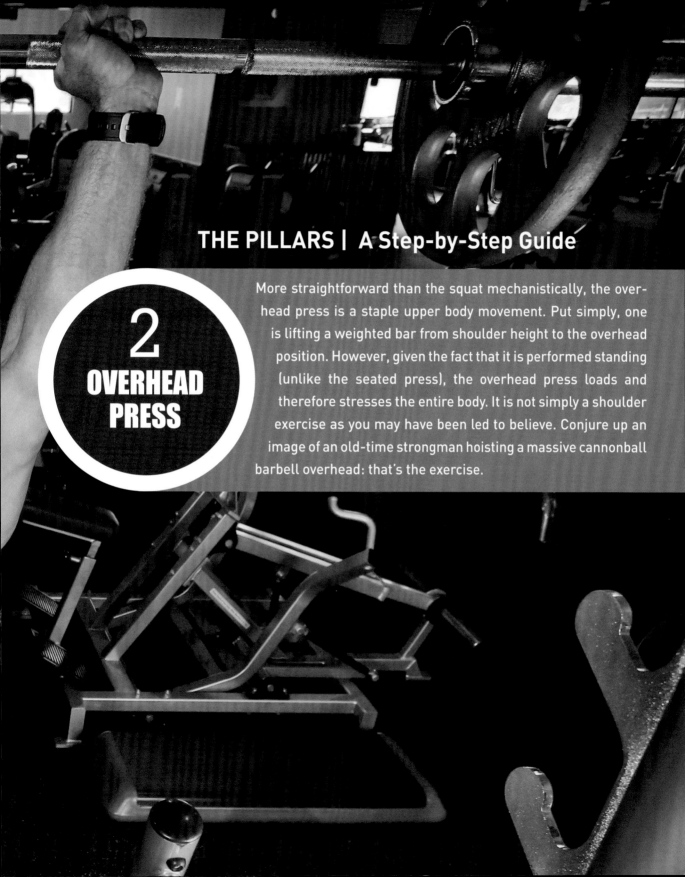

2 OVERHEAD PRESS

More straightforward than the squat mechanistically, the overhead press is a staple upper body movement. Put simply, one is lifting a weighted bar from shoulder height to the overhead position. However, given the fact that it is performed standing (unlike the seated press), the overhead press loads and therefore stresses the entire body. It is not simply a shoulder exercise as you may have been led to believe. Conjure up an image of an old-time strongman hoisting a massive cannonball barbell overhead: that's the exercise.

Overhead presses are contraindicated in trainees with pre-existing shoulder injuries unless medical clearance has been obtained, as the bony elements of the shoulder joint as well as the stabilizing rotator cuff muscles are stressed during the movement.

A thorough warm-up must be performed. This should include active range of motion of the shoulder (including internal and external rotation) and light presses with the Olympic bar (unloaded). Remember, the shoulder is one of the most commonly injured sites among power lifters. By virtue of its anatomy, it is very susceptible to overuse.

To maintain shoulder health and integrity, progress *slowly*, utilizing extreme caution. Gains (after the initial phase of skill learning) will be slow yet steady, as the bench and overhead presses work synergistically.

Driving the bar out of the bottom position of the overhead press. My head and upper torso are slightly rocked backwards to allow the bar to clear the chin (the bar should rest under the chin touching the highest point of the chest at the start position). The elbows are directly under the bar optimizing power transfer in the vertical plane. The abdominal musculature is activated, stabilizing the torso during the movement. There is a subtle form break, though. Do you see it? It is apparent in the next image as well.

OVERHEAD PRESS

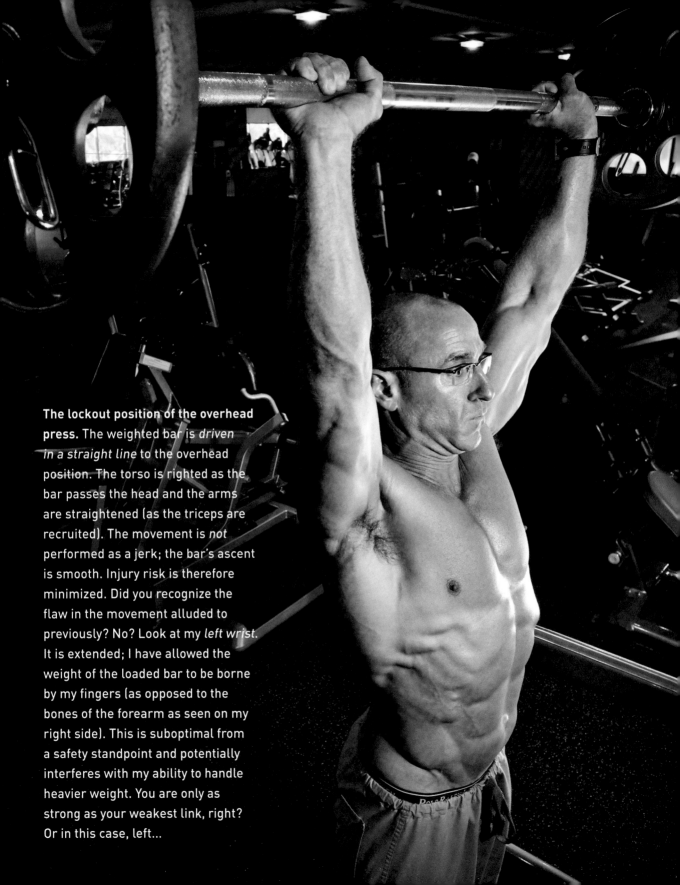

The lockout position of the overhead press. The weighted bar is *driven in a straight line* to the overhead position. The torso is righted as the bar passes the head and the arms are straightened (as the triceps are recruited). The movement is *not* performed as a jerk; the bar's ascent is smooth. Injury risk is therefore minimized. Did you recognize the flaw in the movement alluded to previously? No? Look at my *left wrist*. It is extended; I have allowed the weight of the loaded bar to be borne by my fingers (as opposed to the bones of the forearm as seen on my right side). This is suboptimal from a safety standpoint and potentially interferes with my ability to handle heavier weight. You are only as strong as your weakest link, right? Or in this case, left...

EXERCISE TECHNIQUE

1 Focus on the task at hand. See yourself through the movement before even approaching the weighted bar on the rack. Assure that your spotter is ready.

2 Approach the bar which should be positioned at mid-sternal height. *The bar should abut your mid-high chest.*

3 Grasp the bar (using a forward grip) equidistant from the center knurling (ridges in the bar) in order to establish a *perpendicular* between bar and forearm. This will likely position your hands slightly more than shoulder-width apart. Rotate your elbows forward to assure that they are directly under the bar. This will allow for optimal force transmission to the weighted bar. You are now ready to begin.

4 Unrack the bar by applying subtle vertical pressure through the heel of your palms. *This is not a jerk motion.* It should merely allow you to set the bar into the correct starting position. Specifically, the bar should sit at the low clavicular level (just under the base of the neck). Your forearms should assume a vertical position relative to the bar. If you have done this correctly, you will note your elbows at a 60-70 degree angle *from your body* (0 degrees being straight in front of you). This is your starting position.

5 As dictated by your equipment (cage, rack or stand), carefully take 1-2 steps backwards and steady yourself, feet approximately shoulder-width apart.

6 Inhale, contract your abdominal musculature and press the bar overhead as a single, continuous movement. You will note that your torso tends to rock backwards during the *initial* phase of the press. This is simply the body establishing leverage under the weighted bar by one, aligning the bar with the mid-foot (in the vertical plane) as opposed to the toes (where it rests at the starting position) and two, recruiting the upper chest to assist in the movement. As the bar passes the head during the lockout phase, your torso will typically reassume its vertical position as you inherently attempt to optimize the function of the triceps muscle (activated at the top portion of the movement). *Do not exaggerate this rocking movement. By the same token, it **must** be incorporated into the press, as it allows you to lift heavier weight and thereby stimulate more muscle fiber.*

7 At full triceps extension (lockout), you have completed the positive phase of the overhead press. Exhale.

8 Carefully guide the bar downward to its starting position.

PITFALLS

Excessive lower body contribution to the movement. I have seen it innumerable times. This is not a push press or split jerk. This is an overhead press. The legs are *maintained* slightly bent and serve only as conduits for energy transfer from the ground. This exercise predominantly works the upper body with lower body assist. There is no hip drive as in the squat or deadlift.

Failure to drive the bar vertically via lack of swayback. In the absence of torso swayback, the bar in its ascent to lockout position will potentially strike the face. Swayback therefore allows the bar to clear the face and maintains the vertical path of the bar over the mid-foot, optimizing force transmission. Lacking the appropriate rocking movement, an individual is more likely to drive the bar forward initially in an effort to clear the face. This dramatically reduces the upward force imparted to the bar, reducing one's ability to handle heavier loads. *Optimally, the bar just clears the head in its **vertical** ascent.*

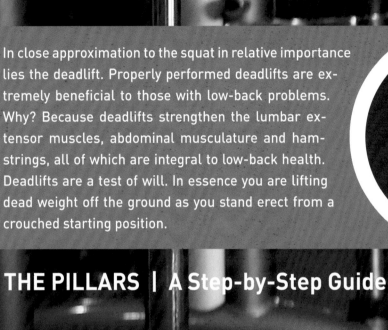

In close approximation to the squat in relative importance lies the deadlift. Properly performed deadlifts are extremely beneficial to those with low-back problems. Why? Because deadlifts strengthen the lumbar extensor muscles, abdominal musculature and hamstrings, all of which are integral to low-back health. Deadlifts are a test of will. In essence you are lifting dead weight off the ground as you stand erect from a crouched starting position.

3 DEADLIFT

THE PILLARS | A Step-by-Step Guide

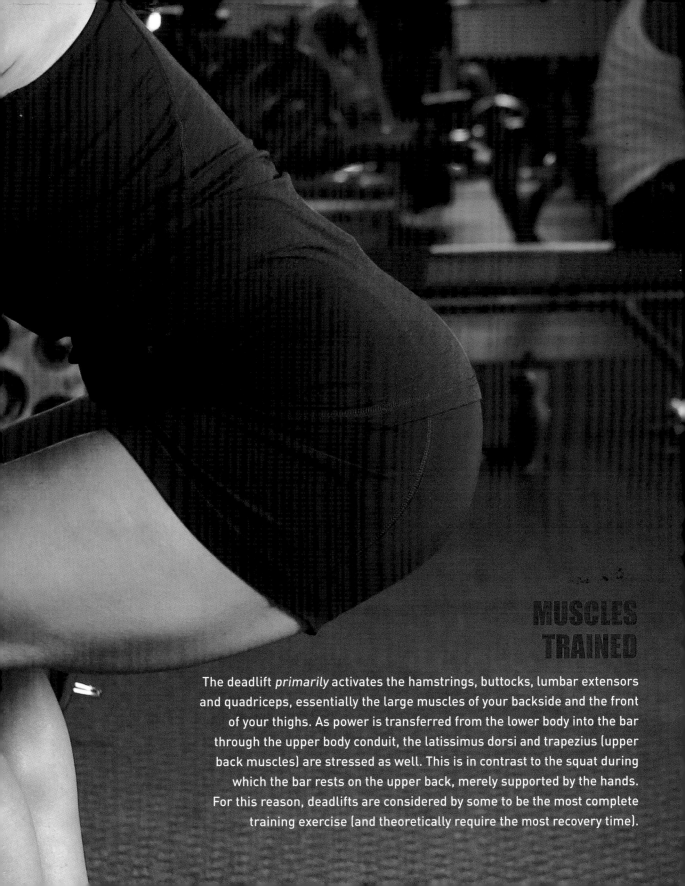

MUSCLES TRAINED

The deadlift *primarily* activates the hamstrings, buttocks, lumbar extensors and quadriceps, essentially the large muscles of your backside and the front of your thighs. As power is transferred from the lower body into the bar through the upper body conduit, the latissimus dorsi and trapezius (upper back muscles) are stressed as well. This is in contrast to the squat during which the bar rests on the upper back, merely supported by the hands. For this reason, deadlifts are considered by some to be the most complete training exercise (and theoretically require the most recovery time).

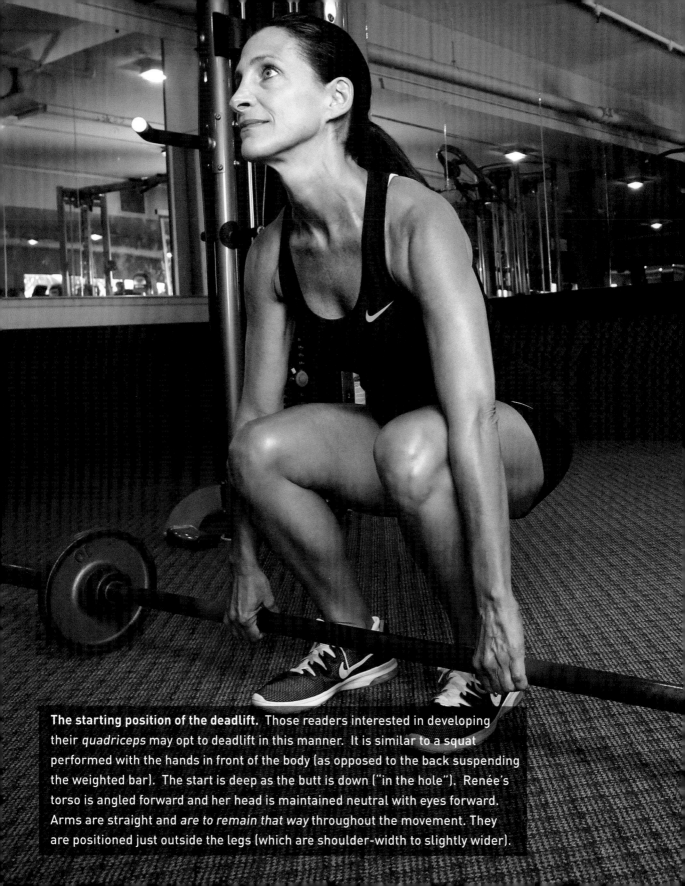

The starting position of the deadlift. Those readers interested in developing their *quadriceps* may opt to deadlift in this manner. It is similar to a squat performed with the hands in front of the body (as opposed to the back suspending the weighted bar). The start is deep as the butt is down ("in the hole"). Renée's torso is angled forward and her head is maintained neutral with eyes forward. Arms are straight and *are to remain that way* throughout the movement. They are positioned just outside the legs (which are shoulder-width to slightly wider).

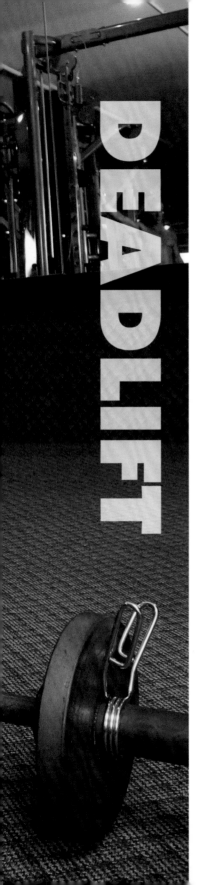

DEADLIFT

IN CLOSE APPROXIMATION TO THE SQUAT IN RELATIVE IMPORTANCE LIES THE DEADLIFT.

Don't panic! I know that many of you were told that deadlifts lead to injury, but this is not so. If that were the case, then why do I prescribe them to my patients who just underwent low back surgery? Properly performed, deadlifts are *extremely* beneficial to those with low-back problems. Why? Because deadlifts strengthen the lumbar extensor muscles, abdominal musculature and hamstrings, all of which are integral to low back health. And this is just one of their many benefits. Similar to squats, deadlifts are not to be neglected. Barring a physical handicap or medical contraindication, *you are not exempt*!

Deadlifts are a test of will. In essence you are lifting *dead* weight off the ground as you stand erect from a crouched starting position. Have you ever seen a demonstration of so-called "proper lifting technique?" That's a deadlift! They stress the entire body and develop functional strength. No longer will you be unable to lift that heavy box off the floor. The strength gained is transferable to activities outside the confines of the gym. Think about it, we have been hoisting loads off the ground and carrying them (more on this later) for eons. The movement pattern is literally etched into our genes. You can't escape it. Don't even try. In fact, embrace it! The hard work will pay off, I promise you....

SAFETY CONSIDERATIONS

Seek the advice of an experienced deadlifter. Learn form and proper technique primarily. This will translate to safety. Do not even consider loading your back with a weighted bar if you have sustained a recent spine fracture or disc herniation, have been diagnosed with osteoporosis or have not been cleared by your doctor (for any preclusive medical condition).

As with squats, you may consider wearing a weight belt to bolster the stability of your low back. I prefer to strengthen the lumbar and abdominal muscles instead, utilizing them as an internal "belt." You may additionally incorporate a Valsalva maneuver to augment the stability of the lumbar spine. This was discussed previously.

Warm-up sets are critical. As the deadlift is a full body movement, both upper and lower body musculature should be appropriately warm prior to deadlift work sets.

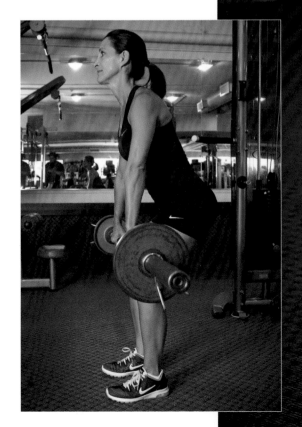

Renée **pulls** the bar up her shins in the vertical plane. The bar *never* lurches forward (which would predispose one to "round-back" lifting and potential injury). Lumbar lordosis is maintained. The initial phase of the movement is performed primarily with her quadriceps. The hamstrings and pelvic musculature are secondarily activated as the pelvis is driven forward (and the hips extended). The arms are held passively at Renée's side. *This is not a row.*

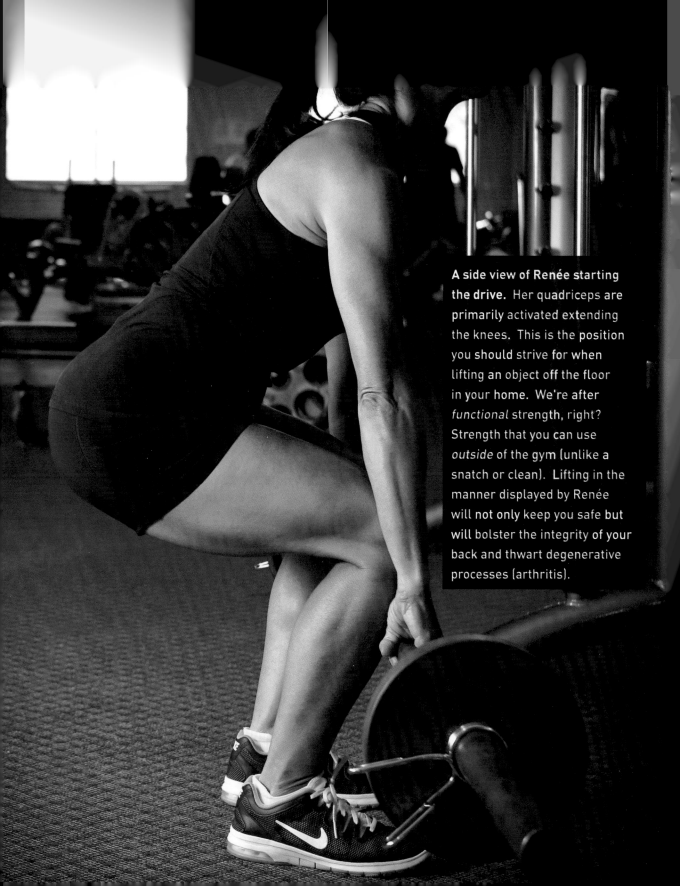

A side view of **Renée** starting **the drive.** Her quadriceps are primarily activated extending the knees. This is the position you **should** strive for when lifting an object off the floor in your home. We're after *functional* strength, right? Strength that you can use *outside* of the gym (unlike a snatch or clean). Lifting in the manner displayed by Renée will **not only** keep you safe **but** will bolster the integrity of your back and thwart degenerative processes (arthritis).

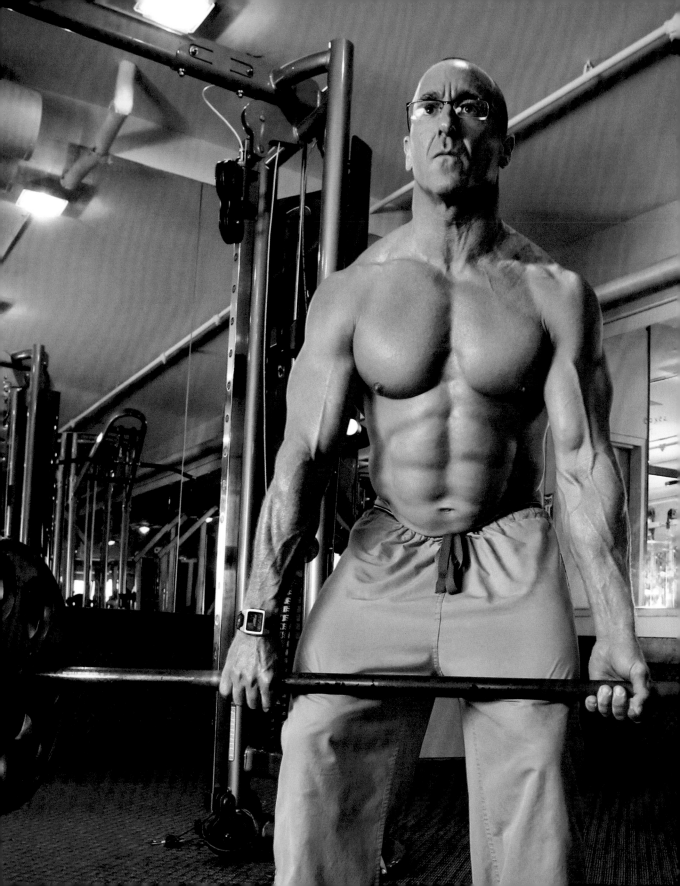

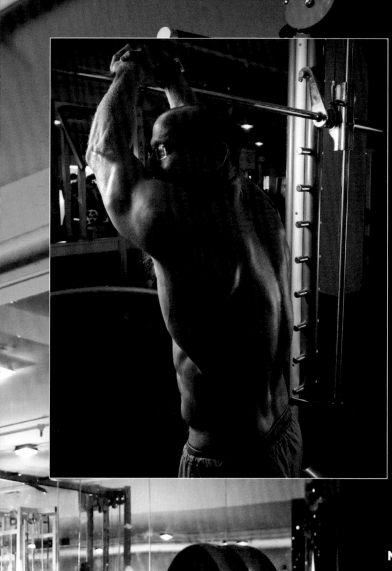

Far Left: Just shy of lockout (when the hips are completely extended). There is activation of the upper torso during the movement but only because it serves as a conduit of the lower body's power. Does this make sense? The bar is not pulled or jerked into lockout. The deadlift is a full body exercise, yes, but *the lower body is the predominant mover* of the weighted bar.

The lumbar musculature serves in a stabilizing role throughout the positive phase and ultimately bears the bar's weight at the top of the movement (when it is least susceptible to injury).

Note:

My deadlifting style assumes that of a powerlifter in that I don't start "deep in the hole" as Renée does. In fact, my hips are held relatively high at the start of the movement. I use my hip extensors to "lever the weight" up as my pelvis is driven forward. This technique is for advanced lifters but can certainly be developed under the supervision of a qualified trainer.

EXERCISE TECHNIQUE

1 Focus on the task at hand. See yourself through the movement before even approaching the weighted bar on the floor. The deadlift, like the squat, is extremely technical.

2 Approach the weighted bar and position your feet shoulder-width apart, feet externally rotated slightly. The bar should be in close approximation to the shins.

3 Grasp the bar just outside the legs with an alternate grip (one hand facing forward and the other backward). This should be performed by flexing forward with straight knees and locked elbows, pre-stretching the hamstrings in preparation for the positive phase of the movement.

4 Allow your buttocks to sink slightly and drive your knees forward until the weighted bar abuts your shins. You will sense tightness in the hamstrings and buttocks (gluteal muscles) which means that these muscles have now been "loaded." This loading is furthered in the next step with the addition of the lumbar extensors.

5 *Without moving your hips,* sway your torso up and back utilizing the lumbar extensor muscles (basically, extend your back). Provided your elbows have remained locked and your arms nearly perpendicular to the ground, you will sense tightness in your low back and latissimus dorsi. The second loading phase is now complete. You are ready to begin the movement as both upper and lower body musculature have been loaded.

6 Inhale. Extend the knees and hips while maintaining the torso angle (established in step #5). *The bar should remain as close as possible to the shins.* In fact, if you haven't marred your shins deadlifting, you simply haven't done enough of them utilizing proper technique. It's simply the cost of doing business.

7 As the bar crosses the plane of the knee, raise your torso by contracting the lumbar extensors. This "co-contraction" with the hip extensors will drive the pelvis and hips forward, completing the positive phase of the movement. Do not shrug your shoulders nor bend your arms to lock the weight out at the top. The arms are passive players and serve only as conduits for power transfer.

8 Exhale. Reverse the process to lower the bar: flex the hips and knees while maintaining a slight arch in your lower back and carefully set the bar on the ground.

PITFALLS

Failure to maintain the bar close to the body

As discussed in the context of other standing movements, the most efficient path for a weighted bar to travel is in a straight line directly over the mid-foot. In order for this to occur, you must engage the latissimus dorsi while elevating the chest during the loading phase and "drag" the bar up the shins during the pull. This takes practice and initially significant concentration. Allowing your shoulders to slump forward, unweighting your heels, or attempting to hoist the weight with your biceps, will potentially shoot the bar forward, diluting your upward force. As in the squat, one's weight during a deadlift should be on the mid-foot and never on the toes. This will predispose you to round-back lifting.

Round-back lifting

As discussed elsewhere, round-back lifting is potentially disastrous to the lumbar spine. Pressure in the intervertebral discs rises significantly when improper round-back technique is employed, predisposing the lifter to a "disc herniation" and a miserable existence.

Maintain a rigid lower back during the ascent. This does not equate to a hyperextended posture. Simply load the hamstrings and buttocks as above and subsequently the low back in order to *establish tension* in the kinetic chain of muscles. Maintain this tension during the pull as you "lever" the weight up.

Poorly synchronized "lever" action of the body

This is by far the most difficult aspect of the deadlift. Follow me here. As the hips are rising during the positive phase of the movement (the direct result of quadriceps activation, i.e. knee straightening), the pelvis is coursing forward and the torso angle is becoming increasingly vertical. This compound movement resembles a lever as both the hips and lumbar spine are rotating into extension about the pelvic axis (which acts as a fulcrum). Any asynchrony during this progression will be manifested as an alteration in bar path (forward or backward) and inefficient force transfer from legs to bar. *Remember, the quadriceps are activated first in the presence of a static torso angle and then the pelvis is driven forward, not the other way around.*

The bench press targets the deltoids (shoulders), triceps and chest *primarily*. As above, there are numerous stabilizing muscles, the largest of which is the latissimus dorsi, that allow for optimal power transfer into the weighted bar. In this regard, do not be surprised if your "lats" are sore after a heavy bench workout. Similarly, as the primary drivers of the weighted bar are the anterior deltoid and triceps, sweat not if your chest is lacking that much sought-after soreness after a heavy session. This is *not* an isolated, bodybuilding-type "chest exercise." Your goal is to deeply inroad the targeted muscles, *in bulk*.

THE PILLARS | A Step-by-Step Guide

Undoubtedly the most popular exercise, the bench press is considered the "benchmark" of an individual's strength, right or wrong. "How much do you bench?" This question seems all too familiar even to novice lifters. Why has the bench press assumed such an important role in our arsenal of exercises? Because it stresses not only the entire upper body but the lower body as well, serving a stabilizing function. Again another *big*, compound, anabolic movement that significantly stresses large muscle groups. *Big* hormonal response. *Big* bang for the buck.

4

BENCH PRESS

And again very basic: while lying on a flat bench, the trainee pushes a barbell off the lower chest until the arms are straight. Sound simple? It is. Remember, there's elegance in simplicity.

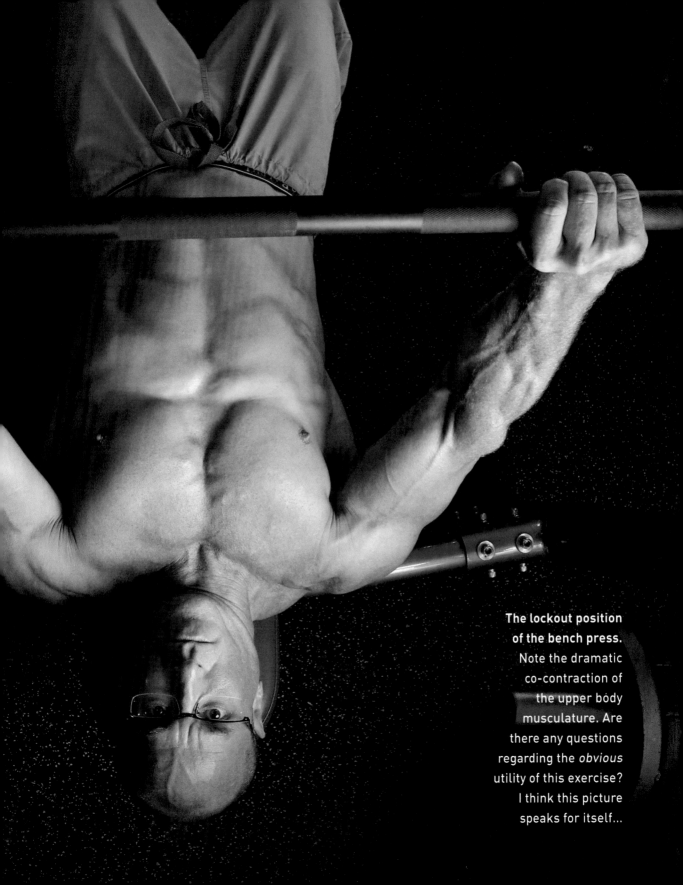

The lockout position of the bench press. Note the dramatic co-contraction of the upper body musculature. Are there any questions regarding the *obvious* utility of this exercise? I think this picture speaks for itself...

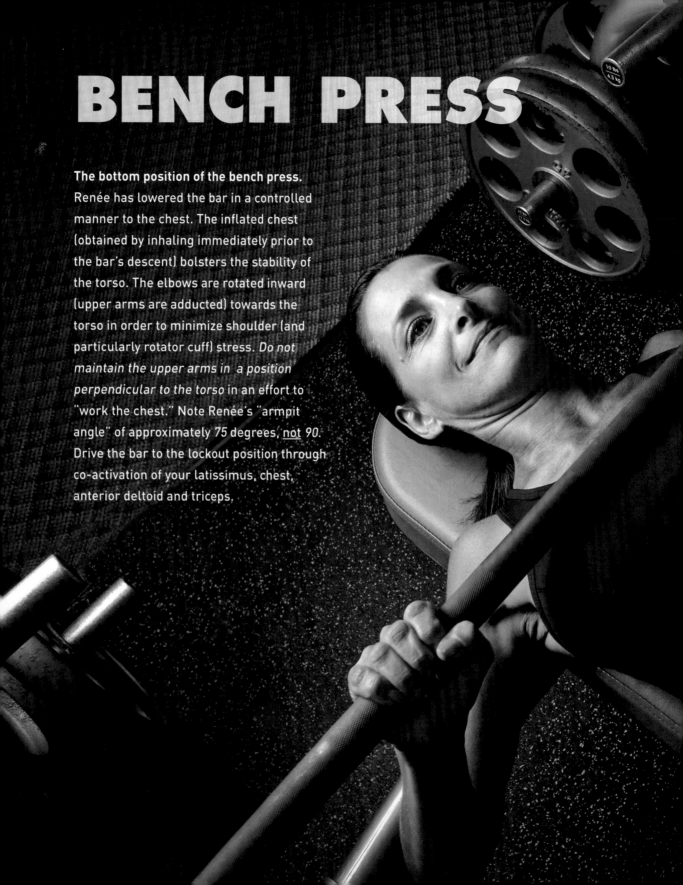

BENCH PRESS

The bottom position of the bench press.
Renée has lowered the bar in a controlled
manner to the chest. The inflated chest
(obtained by inhaling immediately prior to
the bar's descent) bolsters the stability of
the torso. The elbows are rotated inward
(upper arms are adducted) towards the
torso in order to minimize shoulder (and
particularly rotator cuff) stress. *Do not
maintain the upper arms in a position
perpendicular to the torso* in an effort to
"work the chest." Note Renée's "armpit
angle" of approximately 75 degrees, not 90.
Drive the bar to the lockout position through
co-activation of your latissimus, chest,
anterior deltoid and triceps.

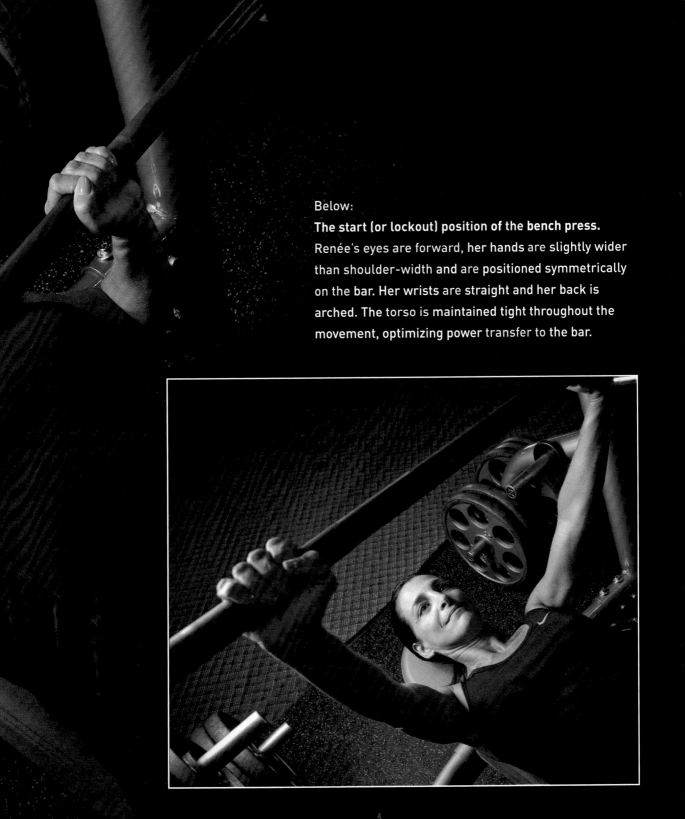

Below:

The start (or lockout) position of the bench press.
Renée's eyes are forward, her hands are slightly wider
than shoulder-width and are positioned symmetrically
on the bar. Her wrists are straight and her back is
arched. The torso is maintained tight throughout the
movement, optimizing power transfer to the bar.

SAFETY CONSIDERATIONS

Learn form and proper technique primarily. This will translate to safety. The shoulder is particularly susceptible to injury *if* improper technique is utilized.

A spotter is mandatory. Don't even consider performing your (heavy) work sets in the absence of a spotter. I have seen people *(and have been)* pinned under a loaded bar. Dangerous and very stupid.

Stated elsewhere, do not neglect your warm-up. I prefer several sets of narrow-width pushups, front (anterior) raises with dumbbells, and bench presses with the unloaded bar.

EXERCISE TECHNIQUE

1 Focus on the task at hand. See yourself through the movement before lying down under the weighted bar.

2 Lie down on the bench. Position your forehead underneath the racked bar. Place your feet flat on the floor.

3 Grasp the bar, hands slightly wider than shoulder-width apart.

4 Arch your back in order to elevate your chest and squeeze your shoulder blades together. The retracted shoulder blades will act as the contact point with the bench and allow for counterforce production (as the body is driven *down* into the bench by the weighted bar).

5 Release the bar from the rack by applying upward pressure into the bar, locking your arms. Allow the bar to course towards the feet until the arms are perpendicular to the torso. *Do not look at your arms in order to confirm the position of the bar.* This correct starting position should be sensed.

6 Inhale and unlock the elbows.

7 In a controlled manner, lower the bar to the *elevated* chest at approximately low-chest level, assuring that your elbows are *below* the plane of your shoulder joint. Stated another way, bring your elbows closer to your body as opposed to flaring them outward during the descent (negative phase). This will markedly reduce the potential for shoulder injury (impingement syndrome). During this lowering phase, attempt to "load" your lats by maintaining tension in them. This must be practiced. Remember, as with the squat, *a solid negative phase primes the involved muscles for a successful drive (positive phase).*

8 Co-contracting the chest, triceps and anterior deltoids (shoulders), drive the bar off your chest. Your wrists and forearms should be in vertical alignment. Maintain an arched back. Apply firm pressure with your feet, yet do not raise your buttocks off the bench. The bar should course *upwards and backwards* in order to reach the lockout position at eye level.

9 Exhale and re-rack the bar with elbows locked and wrists straight.

PITFALLS

Bouncing the bar off the chest. I see this constantly. You are only doing yourself a disservice by rebounding the bar off your elevated chest. For one thing, you are not stressing the target muscles optimally by relying on momentum at the most difficult segment of the movement: the bottom, akin to the "hole" in squats. And secondly, bouncing the bar predisposes one to injury.

Hand in hand with the above is **elevation of the buttocks from the bench.** This is another maneuver utilized to "cheat the weight up." This further elevates the chest off the bench in order to theoretically reduce lockout distance. For the above reasons, this is simply... *stupid.* Ass stays on the bench, back is arched, upper body musculature remains tight throughout the movement, period.

Failure to rotate your elbows downward during the negative phase. This will predispose you to a shoulder impingement syndrome and a foreshortened bench press career. Be sure to rotate your elbows (in) towards your body as the bar descends to your chest. This will also allow for an optimal bar path. Persistently "flared" elbows on the other hand will guide the bar into the upper chest and traumatize your shoulders. Yes, you will potentially obtain a better stretch (and subsequent contraction) of the chest (pectoralis) musculature, but at what cost? The surgical cost of a rotator cuff repair?

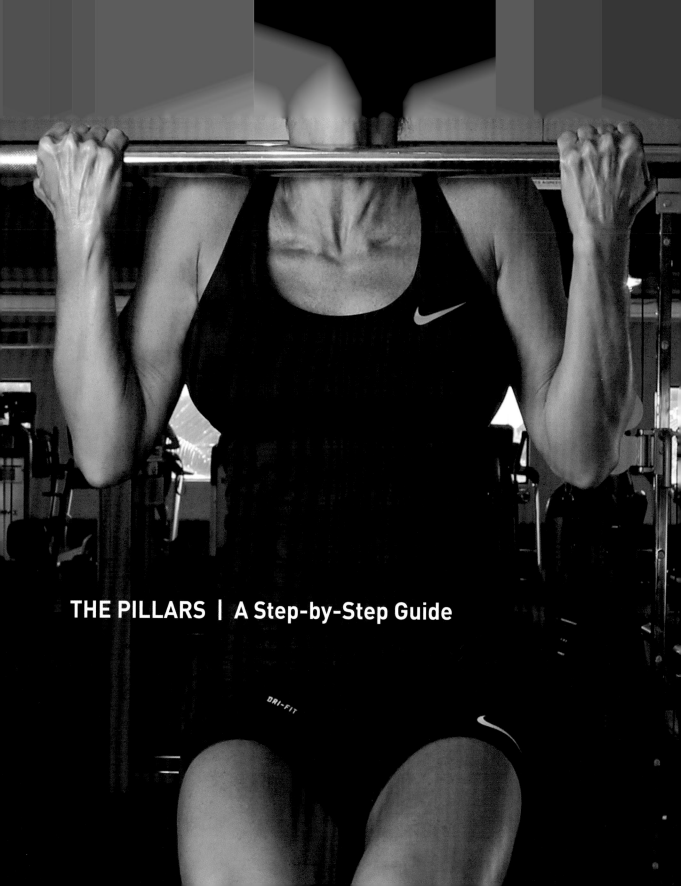

THE PILLARS | A Step-by-Step Guide

The pull-up and chin-up are similar movements and will therefore be addressed as a single unit. The pull-up is performed with a wide overhand grip on the overhead bar and the chin-up with a narrow underhand grip. The **pull-up** stresses the latissimus dorsi primarily while the **chin-up** loads the latissimus and biceps primarily. Both movements also work the accessory muscles of the upper back. The abdominals are stressed heavily during both movements and may be further emphasized by varying leg position (i.e. 'L' position).

5
PULL-UP/ CHIN-UP

Simply one of the most effective exercises out there. Unlike the bench and overhead presses, these exercises stress the upper body musculature that draws loads *into* the body, namely the latissimus dorsi, biceps, rhomboids and rectus abdominis. During a pull/chin-up, one draws the body (the load) towards an overhead bar. Aptly named, the exercise entails doing just that, "*pulling* oneself *up*" from a hanging position.

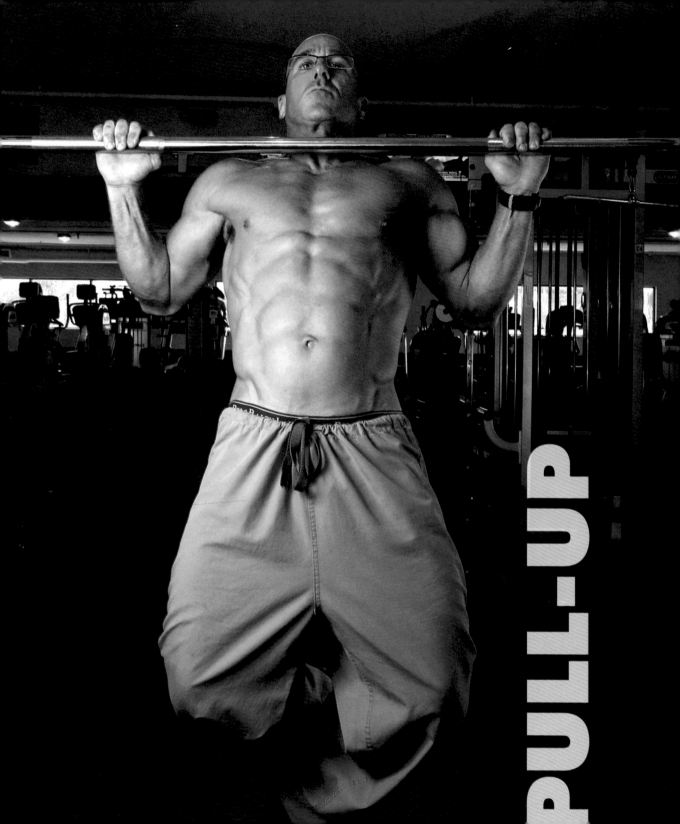

PULL-UP

PULL-UP / CHIN-UP:
Simply one of the most effective exercises out there.

Unlike the bench and overhead presses, these exercises stress the upper body musculature that draws loads *into* the body, namely the latissimus dorsi, biceps, rhomboids and rectus abdominis. During a pull/chin-up, one draws the body (the load) towards an overhead bar. Aptly named, the exercise entails doing just that, "*pulling* oneself *up*" from a hanging position. You've probably heard pull/chin-ups are hard and that 9 out of 10 people can't do one. *Both* statements are true. And there is a reason: Most people simply haven't put forth the effort to acquire the needed strength. Ladies, have you been told that pull-ups are a "man's exercise?" **B.S!** There are no gender-specific exercises. You too *can* and *should* aspire to do consecutive body weight pull-ups. It is well within your capabilities. And you will reap the health benefits of the strength (and muscle) gained in your quest toward that first unassisted pull. Let's get going.

At left: The finish of a **pull**-up. An overhand grip is utilized here. The hands are wider than in a chin-up as this better emphasizes the lats (as does the reduction in biceps involvement accomplished with the grip change). To blast the rhomboids and posterior (back) shoulder musculature, I squeeze my shoulder blades together and stick my chest out (attempting to bring *it* to the bar), in almost a lay-back position. People ask me how I've developed a chiseled abdomen. Well...

At right:
Renée demonstrates a "textbook" finishing position for the chin-up.
And yes, she does them unassisted! In the *chin*-up (as opposed to the
pull-up), an underhand (palms towards the trainee) grip is utilized, and
the hands are spaced slightly wider than shoulder-width. At the finish
(of the positive phase), Renée's chin is well *over the bar*; in fact, the
bar touches the high-chest. This is a manifestation of her strength and
technical prowess. An exercise thought to be out of reach for a female,
chin-ups are *very* doable if you **Get Serious!** Just ask Renée...

SAFETY CONSIDERATIONS

The obvious structure at risk in these movements is the shoulder. It is
placed in a precarious position when one hangs from an overhead bar with
straightened arms. Similarly, the tendons of the triceps and biceps muscles
are stressed during the "hanging" position.

EXERCISE TECHNIQUE

1 Begin by standing under the bar and grasping it either with a wide overhand (pull-up) or narrow underhand (chin-up) grip. Pull-ups are typically performed with a wider than shoulder-width grip and chin-ups with a shoulder-width grip. **Begin with a chin-up** as these are typically easier than pull-ups for most individuals.

2 Grasp the bar with an underhand grip at shoulder-width.

3 Co-contract your biceps and latissimus (back muscles) and attempt to drive your elbows downward as your feet rise from the ground. In the case of a pull-up, your upper arm will be perpendicular to the long axis of your body. Here too, however, you will be attempting to drive your elbows downward.

4 As your body rises towards the bar, lean your head *slightly* backwards to allow it to clear the bar. Maintain a rigid abdomen. Do not be concerned with leg position during this learning period; they will typically fall into position naturally.

5 Complete the positive phase of the movement with continued co-contraction of the biceps, latissimus and rhomboids (muscles between the shoulder blades). Attempt to drive your *chest* into the bar by leaning back and elevating your chest ("showing your feathers").

6 Hold the contracted position for at least a second and then slowly lower your body to the start position.

7 If more repetitions are to be performed, use caution at the extremes of arm extension as noted above.

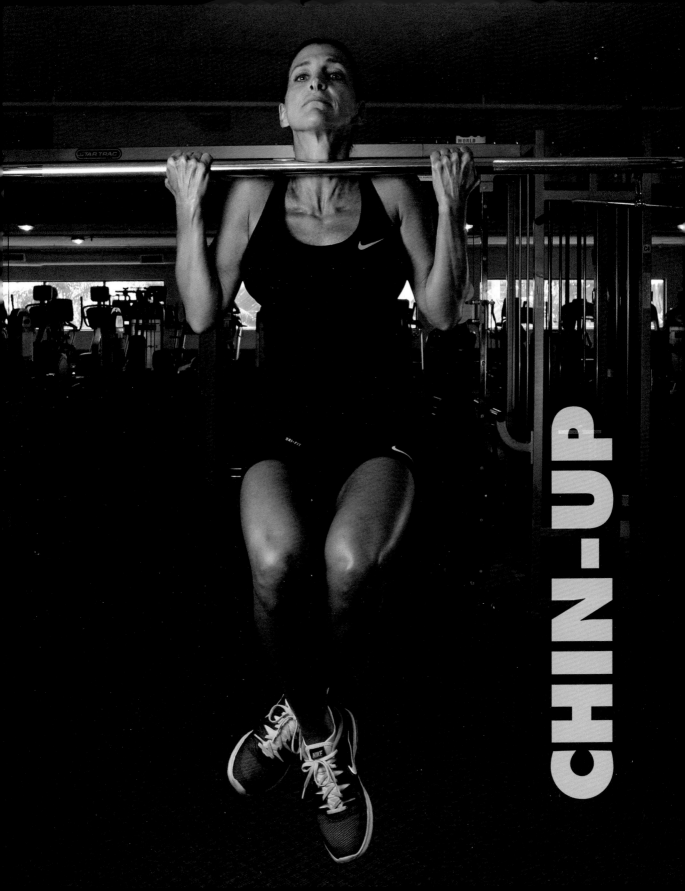

CHIN-UP

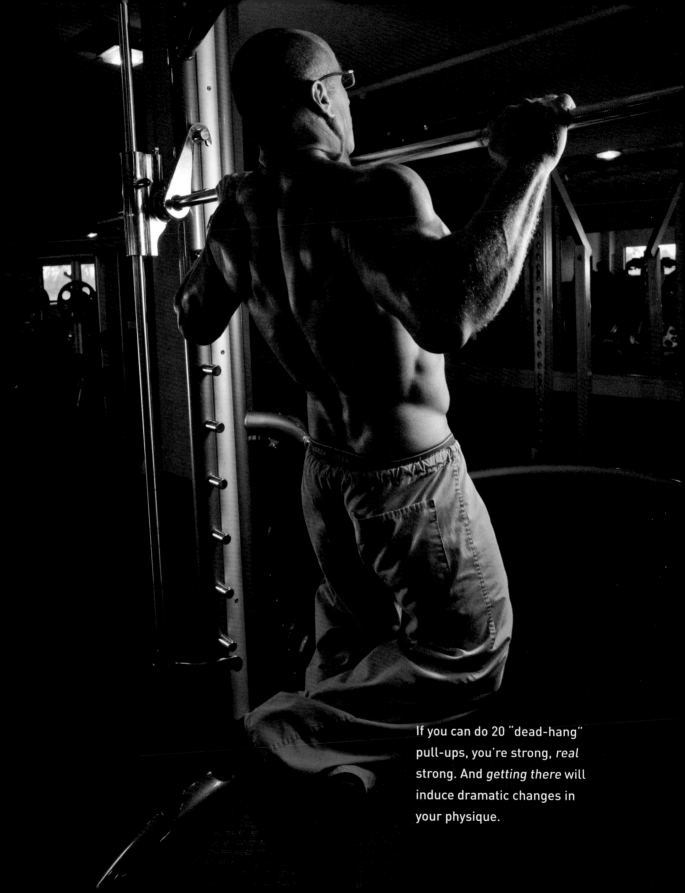

If you can do 20 "dead-hang" pull-ups, you're strong, *real* strong. And *getting there* will induce dramatic changes in your physique.

PITFALLS

Kipping

The bane of my existence. Kipping is a swinging movement of the lower body utilized to drive the upper body over the bar. This deprives you of the benefits of the movement. It is a useless maneuver and has *zero* place in any strength training regimen. Unfortunately, kipping pull-ups are utilized by a variety of "activity-based" workout schemes and have hence become popular. Are the masses by virtue correct? I think not. Skip the kips.

"Rapid-fire" sets with small vertical displacement

If you are going to do a pull-up/chin-up (and we all are, right?), proceed deliberately with proper form. Gym goers often belt out 30 pull-ups with six inches of vertical (up/down) displacement (per rep) in 30 seconds. Worthless. This is a parlor trick. To the uninitiated, it may seem impressive. In actuality, this is nothing more than an endurance feat requiring little strength (particularly in a lightweight individual). If you want to get strong, practice strength not outright silliness to impress the onlookers.

You may be intimidated by even the thought of performing a pull-up. Erase this thought. A pull-up is well within *your* capabilities *if* you are willing to work. The key is a slow progression to your goal in short, truncated steps. And this applies to *any* exercise. In this manner, you will avoid injury and also derive a sense of satisfaction by fulfilling your short-term goals.

At your gym, locate a pull-up/chin-up assist machine (e.g. Gravitron™) and perform sets with maximal assist initially as dictated by the workout protocol (to follow). Begin with chin-ups as they utilize more muscle mass (lats and biceps primarily) and are therefore easier than pull-ups. Gradually reduce the assistance of the machine (over weeks to months) until you are capable of doing reps with minimal or no assistance. See! That was not so bad. In the event that you don't have access to a gym, you may follow a similar graduated program at home (provided you have an overhead bar):

Stand on a raised platform under the bar and perform sets from the elevated platform. Reset your feet on the platform after every rep. After you have completed the prescribed reps per protocol, begin lowering the platform until you have "weaned it off" completely. Congratulations! You have just made significant strides in your level of strength.

This process will take time. As will squatting 315 lbs. to a novice. So even if you start out simply squatting your own body weight, who cares? The benefits of strength training are obtained during your quest for strength. *Throughout your life.* One doesn't one day acquire strength or become "strong." So be patient. Work hard. Avoid injury. Most importantly, don't quit. Persevere. **Claim your health!**

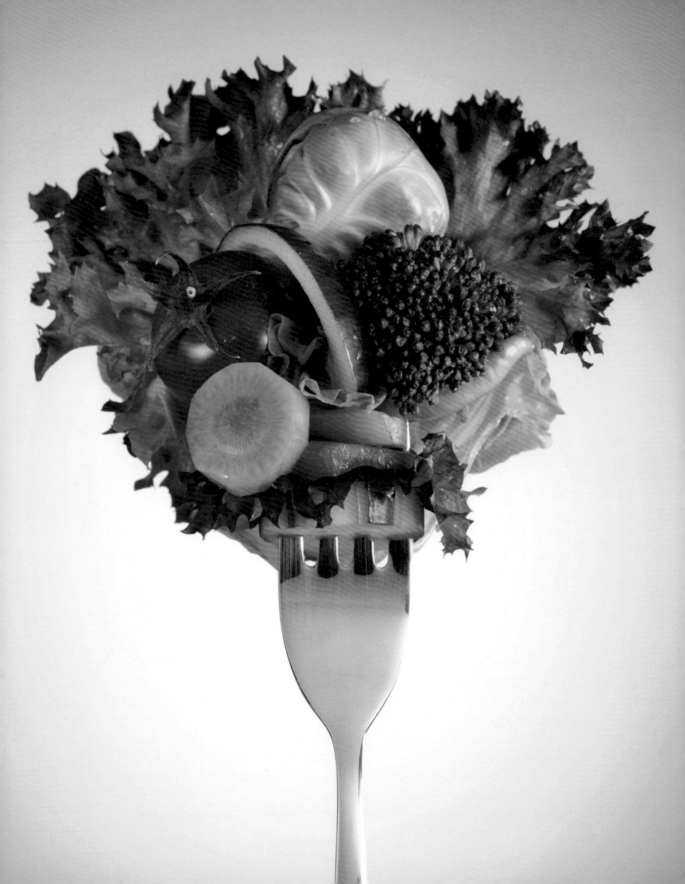

6

FUEL
A BETTER
BODY

This is **NOT** the next diet book. I don't believe in diets. In fact, there is no such thing as a diet. Well-fit individuals were around eons before the word "diet" even existed. In fact, by default—that is, without our own self-destructive behaviors (poor diet and a sedentary lifestyle) the human body is lean muscle. We GROW fat (and fatter) by virtue of our poor lifestyle choices.

Despite the obvious challenges, it was almost easier to stay healthy in Paleolithic times because there was less "interference." There were no supermarkets filled with synthetic, chemically-laden foods. You were hungry, you killed your food, and you picked your fruit and vegetables. And these weren't laced with estrogenic and potentially carcinogenic pesticides. Now it's much more difficult—health takes work. **Requisite to your attainment of health is knowledge.**

While there is some genetic predisposition to gain weight, especially when eating sugars and starches (so-called "carbohydrate intolerance"), you are not *destined* to be fat. So stop blaming your parents. Genetic predispositions can be overcome with diligent adherence to sound nutrition principles. These concepts must be understood in depth *and* at the outset. Education and the resultant knowledge is a prerequisite for execution. Haphazard dieting (there, I said it) in the absence of understanding, will *always* fail in the long run.

Why do I say this? Because sound nutrition (and maintaining a healthy bodyweight) is simply stroking the biochemical processes which are the foundations of our existence as humans. Provide the proper nutrients to *your* biochemistry (which may be slightly different than mine, due to subtle genetic variation) and attain optimal health.

You are a reservoir of biochemical processes, an unbelievably complex machine, albeit with a high degree of predictability. Our bodies, for the most part, act according to a set of rules that evolved over eons as an adaptive response to environmental pressures. Health is attained through sound biochemistry. The absence of health (disease) is biochemical dysregulation. In other words, we start off healthy and we screw it up!

A word to the reader: This chapter is NOT filled with recipes and a meal plan, like most diet books are. It is, instead, filled with information that I think will not only save your life, but give you a good understanding of food and how it works in your body.

More understanding, less memorizing. That way, real-world applications become thoughtless, almost instinctive. You'll make the right food choices without thinking.

My main concern (and it should be your main concern too) is the epidemic of obesity and diabetes in the world, primarily caused by poor diet and lack of activity. Type II diabetes, in particular, is triggered by excess sugary foods that continually require our bodies to produce more and more of the hormone insulin until we ultimately become resistant to its effects, or "insulin resistant." That means our systems are so flooded with this hormone that our cells become immune to its actions, leaving us with high levels of circulating sugar. The excess glucose not only harms our tissues and organs (especially the heart and its feeder arteries), but turns into fat, and turns our bodies into mush instead of muscles. This is the perfect set-up for inflammation which, as I discussed earlier, is at the core of all disease.

Sugar is not the only problem. We consume vast amounts of bad fat which adds fuel to the fire. (Not all fat is equal, which I will explain later.) And we consume too little protein which is essential for building muscle.

Remember, your heart is a muscle too. It—and the arteries that deliver blood to your heart and, ultimately, your body—is especially vulnerable to the toxic effect of high sugar loads and inflammation. Heart disease is still the number one killer of both men and women, so this point is very important.

My goal here is to outline the foundational tenets of nutrition and to present to you the science that will allow you to design your own "diet," one that puts you closer to your fitness goals. Most of you long to shed fat off your waistline. It's really much easier than you have been led to believe. The right food, combined with the right exercise, will get you optimal health and the body you want. First, you need to understand the basics.

As neurosurgeons say to one another, "it's not rocket science." Once you learn all there is to learn, you will see that it's really a common sense approach. You will then be able to make smarter food choices without having to follow a rigid diet.

First Things First: What Is Food?

Food is comprised of three primary nutrients: protein, carbohydrates and fat. Each of these vital nutrients plays a different role in the body. First, you need to understand why we eat, and what food actually does for us.

The purpose of food is to provide us with the building blocks of bodily tissue and the components for ATP (energy) production (essential to keep our hearts beating, our brains thinking, our muscles moving, and our bodies running). Food also serves as a signal alerting our bodies to conditions outside. Think of our food as a liaison between body and environment. When food or certain types of foods are scarce, the body responds in kind. For example, the presence or absence of carbohydrates, through what is known as an "insulin/ IGF-1 signaling pathway," mediates fat storage or breakdown, respectively. In other words, you are telling your body to either burn fat (which you want) or store fat (which often ends up in places where you don't want it). A thorough understanding of this key concept is *vital* to your ability to lose or gain weight. (For example, someone with a wasting disease like cancer needs to know how to conserve body fat and muscle, and even store more. And bodybuilders who want to bulk up also need to know how to add muscle without adding excess fat.)

Elevated levels of serum insulin are suggestive of food surplus, while low levels of insulin signal famine and promote fat breakdown. Remember, these signaling mechanisms have been encoded into our genes to allow us to *adapt* to environmental stimuli. And they are preserved across many species! Just as we produce insulin in response to eating sugar (the stimulus in this case), we produce growth hormone in response to resistance training. Through these signaling proteins (in this case, hormones), the body responds to the state of the external environment. We can utilize this knowledge to our advantage; most of us, however, fail to realize this and succumb to the *very preventable* coronary artery disease, otherwise known as CAD. Remember, "You are only as old as your arteries."

What Are Carbohydrates?

So what about carbohydrates? They've been vilified in recent years, but in reality, our bodies need them, but only the right kind. Basically a carbohydrate is a type of sugar. Molecules of carbohydrate may be linked together (molecules of glucose form glycogen) and stored within the cells. This is known as an insulin-mediated process. As dictated by bodily demand for energy (ATP), the process is reversed and glucose molecules are shuttled into various pathways which ultimately yield ATP.

There are carbohydrates and there are carbohydrates, and therein lies the problem! Broccoli is considered a carbohydrate; so is a lollipop and so is a slice of bread. We all know that vegetables are the far better food choice, yet all of these are carbohydrates. Although very different foods, they provide the substrate for energy-generating biochemical pathways: glucose. Here's the kicker. Carbohydrates are not equivalent to one another. **Complex** carbohydrates are the linked sugar molecules described above and are also known as "starches." **Simple** carbohydrates are single sugar molecules such as glucose, sucrose (table sugar) and fructose. These are termed "sugars" on standard food labels. So why am I telling you this? Because the body's primary *response* to the two types of carbohydrates (the environmental signal) is different, particularly as it relates to insulin secretion from the pancreas.

Glucose molecules are driven into cells in the presence of insulin. This is *independent* of the carbohydrate source (simple or complex, table sugar or broccoli). As dictated by the metabolic demands of the body *at that instant*, glucose is either utilized for ATP production or stored as glycogen or converted to fat. Eat an ice cream sundae and lay on the couch, for example. There is no immediate demand for the consumed glucose and all the surplus is therefore converted to fatty acids and stored as fat. This is why I am an advocate of short walks after a meal; just the opposite occurs. Create a demand and the body will utilize the consumed glucose for energy production, fueling your leg muscles! This equates to less circulating glucose and less AGE formation, in essence conferring protection to the endothelial lining of the blood vessels.

So what happens when you eat a sugar-laden ice cream sundae with a massive amount of simple carbohydrate? These molecules rapidly pass through the lining of the gut and enter the bloodstream, causing extreme elevations in blood sugar. So what *adaptive response* is in place to accommodate this sugar load? Marked elevations in serum glucose can induce coma, but for most of us, this doesn't happen. So how does the body protect itself from this molecular onslaught? What biophysical systems have evolved to accommodate the varying loads of carbohydrates we consume? Blood sugar in healthy individuals is maintained at a relatively constant level despite consumption or lack thereof. The brain is intolerant of extremes of hypoglycemia and hyperglycemia, both of which are associated with **coma**. How is glucose homeostasis maintained? Predominantly through the pancreatic hormone known as insulin.

Insulin is secreted in response to elevations in blood sugar. This process is deranged if not wholly dysfunctional in the type I diabetic (juvenile diabetic). Momentarily, let's consider the inner workings of a healthy individual. Dietary sugar is presented to the system. Pancreatic islet cells in response secrete insulin. Insulin up-regulates receptors on the cell surface which internalize the circulating glucose molecules for storage or ATP production. The sugar in your ice cream sundae is intracellular. You've heard the old adage, "you are what you eat." Well...

This process occurs rapidly in the case of **simple** carbohydrates (i.e. glucose and sucrose); you feel an immediate "sugar high" when you eat a sundae. This is due to the rapid transport of glucose across the intestinal lining and subsequent rise in serum glucose. The process is much more delayed in the context of **complex** carbohydrate ingestion, like when you eat a piece of broccoli. Complex carbohydrates *first* have to be broken down into their constituent monosaccharides (simple sugars) prior to their absorption. Blood glucose rises, albeit at a slower rate. There is no sugar high, and by virtue of this, no "crash." As will be discussed later, the more gradual increase in blood sugar (and lower magnitude of *the* increase) associated with complex carbohydrate consumption is less toxic to the lining of our blood vessels. Why? Several reasons.

Insulin Ups and Down

First, there is less insulin secreted by the pancreas in response to a lower instant-to-instant serum glucose level. Functioning optimally, the pancreas maintains tight control of serum glucose. Blood sugar typically rises to levels < 140 mg/dL and returns to baseline within three hours of a meal (barring a diabetic or insulin-resistant state). In contrast, the pancreas is stressed when exposed to high levels of serum glucose, having to "chase

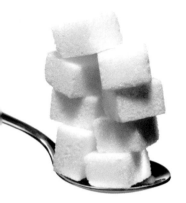

5g of table sugar.
5g of walnuts.
Same weight.

Both have
carbohydrates
with strikingly
different effects
on the body.
In addition,
because of their
high omega-3
content, walnuts
possess anti-
inflammatory
properties.

Sugar? Well you
should know
that by now...

after" the massive sugar attack from the gut. Invariably, insulin levels soar, often overshooting its demand. Therefore, one hour after eating, serum glucose is markedly elevated, as is the level of serum insulin. This occurs even in the context of normal insulin sensitivity, at least until this complex homeostatic mechanism becomes dysregulated, by virtue of chronic bodily exposure to high serum glucose and lack of exercise. You see, high serum glucose in addition to inducing insulin resistance or IR, is toxic to the endothelium, because it promotes formation of "advanced glycation end-products" or AGEs discussed earlier. Glycation is the binding of a glucose molecule to a protein molecule, resulting in the formation of damaged protein structures. Many age-related diseases such as arterial stiffening, cataracts, and potentially Alzheimer's disease, are related to glycation. Cellular accumulation of AGE's induces the production of inflammatory cytokines, which is not good. When you are "over-inflamed," you need to quench the fire.

As a neurosurgeon, I use corticosteroids (powerful anti-inflammatory medicines) fairly aggressively, particularly during the management of a patient with a brain tumor. Having been administered steroids, patients will often report dramatic improvement in not only their headaches, but in their neck and back pain. Why? Because the root of degenerative spine disease, "arthritis," is **inflammation.** Treat the inflammation and the pain improves. Similarly, in the diabetic patient, strategies geared toward diminishing bodily inflammation must be in place. Of course, that is initiated with tight glycemic control.

Know Your GI

You may have heard of the glycemic index (GI) before—it's a way of rating the impact that food has on blood sugar and insulin. In medical terms, GI is defined as the increase in blood glucose level over the baseline level during a two-hour period following the consumption of a defined amount of carbohydrate compared with the same amount of carbohydrate in a reference food. Glucose serving as the reference food has an arbitrarily assigned GI of 100. For the sake of comparison, kidney beans have a glycemic index of 23, peanuts 7, and white rice 89. Simply put, the sweeter the food, the higher the glycemic index or GI value.

Tight glycemic control (finely controlled blood sugar with infrequent, low magnitude spikes) is primarily a function of several different, yet interrelated factors such as ingestion of low glycemic index (GI) foods, lean body mass (particularly in the context of insulin resistance), and daily exercise. There are many other contributing factors such as bodily stress (which may be work-related or due to sleep deprivation). These will be discussed elsewhere.

Why am I telling you this? Haven't myriads of diet books stressed the importance of low glycemic index foods in one's quest to lose weight? You've probably heard it all before, right? Wrong. Yes, low glycemic index carbohydrate consumption facilitates weight loss, but eating your daily vegetables has far greater, life-extending effects. As post-prandial glucose increases only mildly in response to low GI foods, there is less insulin secreted. As insulin is atherogenic and frankly toxic to the endothelium, *lesser* circulating insulin (at any given instant in time) has been correlated with vascular health.

And get this, glycemic fluctuations even within the so-called "normal" range in **healthy** volunteers induce physiologically significant effects on endothelial function, oxidative stress, and immune activation. Even in the **non-diabetic** population, post-meal elevations of plasma glucose exert deleterious effects on the vascular system. I suspect by now you're reconsidering that ice cream sundae! After all, you are likely to die of the effects of atherosclerotic disease or "hardening of the arteries," statistically speaking.

The Real Culprit in Heart Disease

Atherosclerosis—what we know as hardening of the arteries—is not caused by a high fat diet as was once speculated. Let me clarify that, a high fat diet *in the context of* low carbohydrate consumption is **not** atherogenic. Case in point is the Atkins high fat/low carb diet. A 2004 entry in the Annals of Internal Medicine (among many other studies) documents such an effect. The study cohort, comprised of 120 overweight hyperlipidemic individuals, was subjected to either a low-carbohydrate or low-fat diet. Effects on body weight, body composition, fasting serum lipid levels, and tolerability were assessed at 24 weeks. At the outset, one would assume that the subjects on the low-fat protocol would exhibit greater improvements in their lipid profile than those in the low-carbohydrate (and *relatively* high fat) group. After all, eating fatty foods must increase your triglycerides, right? Wrong. Why? Because those on the low carbohydrate diet were *existing* in a low-insulin state. Continuously. The primary stimulus for insulin release, carbohydrate, had been eliminated. And as insulin is a significant stimulus for triglyceride synthesis, its relative absence in those patients on low-carbohydrate diets resulted in significantly **reduced** triglyceride levels. And this lipid-lowering effect was more pronounced in the low-carbohydrate cohort than in the low-fat (*relatively* high-carbohydrate) subjects. In addition, serum inflammatory markers are also reduced on such diets. This last point is crucial. Why? **Because lowered circulating insulin results in lowered bodily inflammation, equating to lower disease incidence and slowed aging.**

Yes, we are all capable of modulating the aging process through sound nutrition, of lowering disease incidence simply by watching what we put in our mouths, particularly as it relates to the **sugar** content of our food. (Note the word "carbohydrate" was purposely excluded from the last sentence. Why? Because not all carbohydrates are bad; they are vital to our health, in fact.)

As you certainly have gleaned from the discussion on glycemic index, a carbohydrate is not a carbohydrate, **is not a carbohydrate!** 5 grams of ingested table sugar induces significant elevations in serum glucose *and* a parallel rise in insulin levels (to accommodate the glucose load). Both the glucose and insulin are toxic to the endothelium, pro-inflammatory and therefore bad for your heart, resulting in elevated oxidative stress. Chronic exposure to such high GI carbohydrates is associated with the development of type II diabetes and heart disease.

In contrast, low glycemic index carbohydrates or those with scores between 0 and 50, exert more salubrious effects on the vascular tree and other bodily systems. The same 5 grams of *walnuts*, for example, has a GI of 15 and because of their high omega-3 content, exert anti-inflammatory and other protective effects on the body. Table sugar. Walnuts. Same weight. Differing carbohydrates. And very different signals as interpreted by the body. One deters the aging process, the other places you one step closer to the reaper. High glycemic index carbohydrates, except in the post-workout recovery period, should be limited.

What About Protein?

Insulin is not only secreted in the context of blood sugar elevations, but it is also secreted in the presence of amino acids, the building blocks of proteins. Amino acids are assimilated into muscle, our protein storage depot. Glucose is ultimately converted into fatty acids and stored as adipose tissue (fat). *Both* occur under the influence of insulin, as it is an **anabolic** hormone.

Anabolism is defined as the constructive phase of metabolism characterized by the conversion of simple substances into the more complex compounds of living matter.

Anabolic processes require energy. That stored or "potential" energy (within the assimilated fatty acid or protein structures) may be called upon in the future, during periods of starvation for example. Amid such **catabolic** (starvation) states, the process of anabolism is reversed as tissues are broken down into their building-block substrates and ultimately released into the bloodstream. Lipolysis, or fat breakdown, is such a process; it is energy-releasing. Adipose tissue is catabolized to fatty acids during steady state endurance exercise or "cardio." Why? To provide substrate for the biochemical reactions that produce ATP or energy. The stored energy in bodily fat is harnessed via a process known as beta-oxidation. Why do you think endurance athletes typically have low body fat percentages? Because type I muscle fibers (those heavily stressed during bouts of endurance exercise) primarily oxidize or burn fatty acids to produce ATP, which ultimately fuels the contraction mechanism.

Too much body fat can be very dangerous. It was once thought that fat or adipose tissue was simply an idle depot for energy storage. Recent data suggest a more sinister role. Adipose tissue functions as an organ by secreting chemical messengers known as adipocytokines, most of which are pro-inflammatory in nature. Extrapolating, the fatter you are, the greater the level of bodily inflammation and likelihood that you will develop type II diabetes. This is in stark contrast to muscle, which serves a protective role with potentially life-extending properties.

Muscle Is Critical

Muscle allows us to move, lift heavy objects, and maintain our upright posture. Of equal importance, however, is muscle's role as *the* protein reservoir for the body. About 40 percent of the body weight of a healthy human adult (weighing about 150 pounds) is muscle, which is composed of about 20 percent muscle protein. Thus, the human body contains about 11 to 13 pounds of muscle protein. This source of protein can be utilized in the nutrient-deprived state to maintain plasma levels of amino acids (for uptake by other organs) and via a process known as gluconeogenesis, to maintain blood *glucose* in the normal range. Yes, the amino acid constituents of protein can be utilized to generate glucose during times of starvation and low-carbohydrate intake.

Muscle protein is essential because it is called upon to service the needs of the body during periods of stress. The stressed state, such as that associated with sepsis, cancer, and traumatic injury, imposes significant demands on bodily protein stores for the provision of amino acids. These precursors are utilized for the synthesis of acute phase reactants, immunoglobulins (antibodies), and those proteins involved in wound healing. Accordingly, cancer survival rates, and survival rates for most injuries, are significantly worse in patients with reduced lean body mass. And this is one of the many reasons that an elderly patient fares poorer than a young one with an equivalent bodily insult. There is simply less reserve. **Our reserve, our resilience to illness, lies in our muscle.**

Motor function aside, muscle serves a crucial metabolic role as well. In other words, muscle burns more calories and fat, which produces a sleeker, stronger, more attractive body. Muscle also increases insulin sensitivity, which helps protect against diabetes.

Muscle, in addition to being a storage depot for protein, also stores significant amounts of glucose in the form of glycogen. Why? As discussed earlier, glucose is a substrate for ATP production. ATP fuels muscle contraction. The relatively large quantities of stored glycogen (1200 kcal), to a great degree, account for the muscular *size* of bodybuilders, as each gram of glycogen is stored with three grams of water. As table salt "attracts" water, glycogen does similarly, literally sucking water into the muscle. Glucose uptake and glycogen assimilation occurs under the influence of...

Insulin, of course.

What Insulin Does

Insulin regulates blood glucose levels by signaling cellular GLUT receptors to migrate onto the cell surface. These complex cell membrane proteins internalize glucose molecules for storage or immediate conversion to ATP. Blood glucose is accordingly lowered. Glucagon, another pancreatic hormone, serves the opposite function, elevating circulating glucose levels. These two hormones in addition to cortisol, norepinephrine (noradrenaline), and growth hormone maintain blood sugar levels within normal limits (70-99 mg/dL).

There is dysregulation of this homeostatic process in the insulin resistant patient. Chronic blood sugar elevations, among other inciting factors, cause a "desensitization" of cells to the presence of insulin. Insulin resistance un-checked ultimately progresses to type II diabetes. The majority of type II diabetics are overweight or obese (as per BMI classification). In such individuals, there is a paucity of muscle or metabolically active tissue *relative* to fat. Lean body mass is simply lacking. And the presence of fat, by virtue of its secretion of adipocytokines, perpetuates the cycle of insulin resistance, as more and more insulin is secreted in response to the increasing fat mass. *Insulin resistance is a resistant disease, period.* But you can break the cycle! How?

Through the addition of muscle mass and loss of body fat. Remember, muscle is metabolically active tissue. During bursts of activity, glucose is the preferred fuel for ATP generation. While a portion of this substrate comes from local intramuscular sources (glycogen), glucose may be drawn into the myocyte (muscle cell) from adjacent capillaries to accommodate metabolic demands. Serum glucose is tapped in essence. This increase in skeletal muscle glucose uptake during exercise probably results from a coordinated increase in rates of glucose delivery (higher capillary perfusion), surface membrane transport, and intracellular substrate flux through glycolysis. Basically, there is an intracellular glucose deficiency that has to be replenished in order to meet the metabolic demands of the muscle, and this occurs concomitantly through several mechanisms. Keep in mind that such rapid influx of glucose occurs predominantly in *type II* or *fast-twitch* muscle fibers, as they rely predominantly on glucose for ATP production (either via aerobic or anaerobic glycolysis).

What does this mean to you? Well, in order to rapidly drive glucose into muscle cells, you must create *the* intramuscular glucose deficiency described above. How? Through intense resistance training. Not "cardio" (should be a four-letter word). This may take the form of high-intensity, strength-endurance type training, such as rowing or cycling intervals, or classic-type hypertrophy training (8-12 reps per set). There will be more on this later. The muscles synthesized in response to such training (type IIa and type IIb fibers predominantly) will serve as "glucose sinks" during *and* between workouts, within the recovery period. The metabolic benefit therefore is **longstanding**. This is in stark contrast to that derived from endurance (steady state) training. As no muscle is synthesized in response to such training, there is little metabolic benefit post-workout. The "fat burn" is *during* the training session.

Muscle fiber hypertrophy regardless of fiber type requires adequate protein intake. This will allow (and promote) the synthesis of contractile proteins, actin and myosin. In the absence of adequate recovery substrate, even in the context of proper training (the stimulus for muscle growth), hypertrophy will not occur. In fact, you may fall victim to overtraining and muscle loss (via catabolism)!

So How Much Protein Is Enough?

This has been a topic of much debate in recent years. There are countless articles in strength and bodybuilding journals, all of which recommend an augmented protein intake to promote muscular recovery. After all, resistance training is elective trauma to the muscular structures. It is this damage which serves as the external stimulus to which the body adapts *by* accumulating muscle mass. And this anabolic process must be supported with adequate protein intake. That being said, adequate protein intake does not mean RDA levels of protein intake (.8g/kg)! The RDA in general is an absolute joke, far underestimating the true needs of individuals, especially those of us assuming the physiologic impact of multiple stressors, let alone training. Such bodily stresses deplete our bodily stores of precise micronutrients. Yet the RDA for vitamin C is 90 mg (for the adult male). I don't know about you, but I'd prefer *not* to live on the threshold of scurvy. Diminishing protein stores (e.g. muscle atrophy) that occur as a by-product of an unchecked aging process account, to a great degree, for the frailty and susceptibility to disease seen in the elderly population.

So what's the verdict? How much protein is enough? Again, I default to the science. According to Tipton et al, protein synthesis in the recovering muscle can be maximized with approximately 15g of orally amino acids administered in the post-workout period. Extrapolating, Co-author Robert Wolfe, PhD opines:

"The response to a single dose of amino acids can be potentially achieved multiple times per day, with additive effects, with repeated meal ingestion. Consequently, it would not be unreasonable to expect beneficial effects stemming from increased myofibrillar and mitochondrial protein synthesis to be achieved with the ingestion of 15g essential amino acids at each meal rather than at only one meal per day. This would equate to a protein intake as high as 1.8g per kilogram per day."

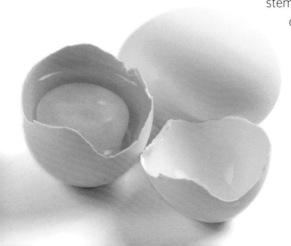

And there you have it. Bottom line, in English. Optimize the physical and metabolic function of muscle by eating 0.8 g of protein per pound of bodyweight daily. Accordingly, a 75 kg (individual would ideally consume 132 g (75 kg x 2.2 lbs/kg x 0.8 g protein/lb) of protein per day. Erring on the cautious side to assure positive nitrogen balance (protein synthesis > breakdown), one would consume **1g protein/lb of bodyweight**. Simple, easy to remember, yet easier said than done. Health takes work, remember!

Naysayers among you are thinking, "I don't need all that protein to gain muscle" or "that amount of protein will damage my kidneys." With regard to the first, always err on the side of surplus protein consumption (as per the above calculation). It is unlikely that the added protein calories (4 kcal/g of protein) will affect body fat levels in a detrimental manner. In fact, quite the opposite often occurs. So bolster your protein intake for a leaner you!

And don't hesitate to do so unless specifically instructed by your physician to do otherwise. Would eating several chicken breasts daily damage your kidneys? Get Serious people. Some bodybuilders eat 500g of protein daily. Are they on dialysis? Umm... No.

So if you are going to make *any* changes to your current nutrition regimen, default to upping your protein intake (provided there are no medical contraindications to doing so). Bodybuilder or not, protein is your best friend, offering a myriad of health-enhancing benefits.

The Best Sources of Protein

Bodybuilders (who, during contest season eat extremely cleanly) mostly obtain their protein from fish, chicken and eggs. Typically dairy (milk and cheese) is shunned by virtue of its *suspected* estrogenic properties, and therefore its tendency to promote body fat storage. And while American skim milk appears to have low levels of hormones (as they are typically resident in milk fat), soy milk has estrogenic *properties*, in addition to being a fairly potent allergen. My personal recommendation would be to avoid soy milk as a protein source in favor of the others. If you are inclined to eat dairy as I am, choose lactose-free (enzymatically treated) low-fat cottage cheese. A typical 1/2 cup serving contains 80 kcal, 1g of fat, 7g (3g sugar) of carbohydrate and 12g of protein. Vegetarians, regimen permitting, may obtain their protein from eggs, low-fat cottage cheese, legumes, walnuts, and almonds. Be aware, however, of the caloric content of nuts. As they provide a significant amount of so-called "healthy fats," nuts are calorically dense, and consumption must therefore be limited in those individuals wishing to shed body fat.

Some Fat Is Good

But is all fat bad? The mere word evokes unpleasant images, carrying with it a very negative connotation. Is this warranted? Or is this just a big misunderstanding? Formerly, fat was regarded as metabolically inert storage tissue accessible during times of starvation. More recently, however, scientists have learned that *stored* fat, particularly visceral fat (that which surrounds the organs as opposed to that lying beneath the skin), serves a more sinister function, the perpetuation of insulin resistance. So fat is bad, right? Wrong. Fat is an absolute necessity for life. The membranes that surround our body's cells are predominantly lipid (fat), and the brain is nearly 60 percent fat! The integration of such fats, particularly the omega-3 fatty acids, into the brain is critical for development during fetal and post-natal periods. Myelin, the encapsulating material that serves as "insulation for the nerves," is composed of DHA, an omega-3 fatty acid. This sheath is disrupted via an autoimmune process (the body attacking itself) in diseases such as multiple sclerosis, appropriately categorized as a "de**myelin**ating disease." This results in impaired neural transmission and, at times, severe neurologic debility. My point is... we **need** fats!

All Fats Are Not Created Equal

If this seems paradoxical, that I've contradicted myself, let me explain. All fats were not created equally. You may have heard that there are "good" and "bad" fats. This is true. But I want you to understand *why*.

So-called "bad" fats are unfortunately those consumed mostly in America. This *partially* accounts for the 30 percent obesity rate in this country and our lower than expected (given our advancements in medicine) longevity relative to countries worldwide. Yes, USA ranks an embarrassing 22nd among developed countries. Don't blame Burger King or McDonald's if you are obese. Blame yourself for making poor food choices. Too much "bad" fat and (equally bad) high glycemic carbohydrate consumption is the proverbial recipe for disaster, the genesis of **most** modern-day diseases and accelerated aging. They feed off one another if both are presented to the body in a single sitting. Why? You should know better by now: insulin and the oxidative stress associated with the consumption of sugar-laden foods. "Bad" fats in this unfriendly, malignant milieu become even more toxic to the vascular endothelium. Again, you are only as old as your arteries.

The most common stratification scheme, the one used on food labels, categorizes fat according to the degree of "saturation." There are saturated and unsaturated fats. Trans fats, also displayed, are synthetic versions of unsaturated fats that were designed to add taste to foods, yet possess disastrous health consequences. For purposes of discussion, the biochemical structures of these fats and, henceforth, the nomenclature are unimportant. What I want you to understand, however, is that *both* saturated and unsaturated fats are essential to health. Saturated fats? Wait. Aren't those bad for us? Not as bad as was once thought. Ironically, their cautious consumption may confer protection against a variety of diseases. On the other hand, unsaturated fats are not all "good." Omega-3 fatty acids isolated from cold water fish, yes; omega-6 fatty acids in the context of the American diet, no. Allow me to explain...

Saturated Fat Is Not Always Bad (or always good)

Saturated fats have been demonized in recent years. As saturated fats are typically solid at body temperature, logic would suggest that saturated fats are the "artery clogging" agents of atherosclerotic disease and are therefore to be avoided like the plague. Not so fast! And certainly not so simple. Saturated fats serve a variety of critical biologic functions such as protein activation, maintenance of cell membrane rigidity, and induction of apoptosis (programmed cell death) in cancer cells. Secondly, atherogenesis is an extremely complex process related more so to oxidative stress and inflammation than a particular subset of fat. As a result, the notion that saturated fat in isolation *causes* atherosclerosis is simply an untruth.

And here's why. Saturated fat *in the presence of* high glycemic index carbohydrates, or reduced levels of "good" polyunsaturated fats, elevates LDL or "bad" cholesterol levels. On its own, it doesn't.

My point? You *can* eat saturated fat, and in fact *need* to. Saturated fats are integral to a variety of physiologic processes, some of which are protective in nature. Consider the study performed by Krauss, *et al* which quantified the effect of dietary carbohydrate and saturated fat on LDL particle size, a major determinant of atherogenic potential. In the context of the low carbohydrate diet, high dietary saturated fat was associated with increases in large, but not with small, LDL, relative to diets with a lower saturated fat content. It's true! Saturated fats when consumed as part of a low carbohydrate diet are associated with **reduced** atherogenic potential of LDL.

You must be thinking, "Why can't I eat loads of saturated fat then? It reduces the effects of "bad" cholesterol, right?" Right, but only under favorable conditions. Low insulin levels are mandatory as is high dietary omega-3 fatty acid intake. Unfortunately, the typical American diet fosters high insulin levels, lacks adequate omega-3 fatty acids, and is replete with omega-6 fatty acids, which in excess are inflammatory in nature. This milieu is atherogenic or artery-clogging!

Why the French Can Eat Pâté and Not Die!

It is becoming increasingly apparent, however, that **the environment into which potentially "bad" fats are introduced is far more important than their actual consumption**. Enter the French Paradox, the observation of low coronary heart disease (CHD) death rates despite high intake of dietary cholesterol and saturated fat. Some have ascribed this lowered incidence to the antioxidant properties of red wine, others to the "Mediterranean" diet. And this effect was similarly noted in the Lyon Diet Heart Study:

Adoption of a Mediterranean style diet that included an increased intake of the omega-3 fatty acid alpha-linolenic acid, a reduction in saturated fat to 8 percent compared with 11.7 percent of energy, and a modest increase in fiber and total carbohydrate was associated with a 72 percent reduction in recurrent coronary events in individuals with a previous heart attack.

As the details of this pronounced effect continue to elude the scientific community, I wouldn't lose too much sleep over its complexities. Understand that it works nevertheless, and utilize this knowledge! *Create a favorable internal environment through sound nutrition, by limiting refined sugars and increasing consumption of both dietary fiber and omega-3 fatty acids.* Saturated fat, should you wish to indulge in that dark chocolate bar, will be much better tolerated in this context, and in fact may be good for you!

Omega-3 Fatty Acids: The Best Fats

As you may have surmised by now, omega-3 fatty acids serve a protective role in the body. Omega-3 fatty acids, like omega-6 fatty acids, are considered **un**saturated fats because of the presence of "double-bonds" in their molecular structure. This renders a degree of flexibility or slipperiness. They are, therefore, oils at room temperature unlike saturated fats, which are predominantly solid (Crisco anyone?). The presence of the double bond also confers a degree of reactivity to unsaturated fats. Through a series of enzymatic reactions, these fatty acid substrates are converted to chemical signaling molecules, the so-called "eicosanoids." Those derived from omega-6 fatty acids are generally pro-inflammatory (induce bodily inflammation), while those from omega-3 fatty acids are much less so and even possess *anti-inflammatory* properties. Please don't misinterpret this last statement. Both omega-3 and omega-6 fatty acids are essential to life, so don't establish a moratorium on the latter; you'll die (really).

By now you should be asking yourself, "Why do I need to eat omega-6 fats if they make my body inflamed?" And the answer relates directly to balance. Think about it. Your body *needs* inflammation, but for discrete periods of time *only*, to fend off disease and repair tissue (muscle electively injured during a workout, for example). *Long-term* inflammation is a primer for disease. Remember the association between gingival disease and atherosclerotic heart disease? *Every* disease, yes *every* disease, possesses an underlying inflammatory component. This is foundational, and paramount to your understanding of aging and age-related disease (from which we are statistically likely to die). **Squelch inflammation and by doing so, retard the aging process.**

Omega-6 fatty acids, specifically linoleic acid, may be obtained from vegetables, nuts, and seeds. Yes, this is why a daily serving of almonds or walnuts is good for you! As most Americans consume a surplus of omega-6 fatty acids relative to protective omega-3 fatty acids, the respective biochemical pathways are driven preferentially (and dangerously) toward formation of arachidonic acid and subsequently prostaglandin E2. Therein lies the genesis of bodily inflammation, better termed inflamm-**aging**. Diabetes, mechanistically, is an inflammatory disease. See why? Because the excess sugar facilitates bodily production of arachidonic acid. The flames of inflammation, and the persistent oxidative stress associated with elevated blood sugars, accelerate the atherogenic process. Take a guess what these patients die from.

Vascular disease! Simply put, diabetics die of complications related to atherosclerotic occlusive disease, *at an early age*. They die of accelerated aging. For this reason, in addition to tight glycemic control, diabetics must dramatically increase their intake of omega-3 fatty acids. And YOU should too, independent of your existing medical problems! Strive for an omega-6:omega-3 ratio of 1:1. Protect your body with anti-inflammatory omega-3 fatty acids, in high doses, as statistically speaking, your diet is suboptimal.

A Little Omega-6 Goes a Long Way

Yes, unlike the Japanese, Americans consume excessive amounts of omega-6 fatty acids. In fact, our consumption of soybean oil has increased a thousand-fold in the last century. Soybean oil has a markedly unfavorable omega-6:omega-3 of 7:1. Remember, an ideal ratio is 1:1. It should be of no surprise to you then that disease incidence has risen in parallel with our consumption of these inflammatory *foods*. Yes, foods. Not to sound cliché, but there is some truth to the saying "you are what you eat." Both omega-3 and omega-6 fatty acids are incorporated into cellular membranes as *phospholipids*. In fact, the cell membrane is a storage depot *for* fatty acids from which the various prostaglandins are derived. And while small amounts of omega-6 fatty acids are essential to the body, high concentrations within the cell membrane *from* excess consumption are causally related to bodily inflammation and more specifically, chronic disease. Why? Again, the increase in arachidonic acid (an omega-6 fatty acid derived from the metabolite DGLA) leads to an increase in pro-inflammatory prostaglandins and a decrease in those derived from EPA/DHA (omega-3 fatty acids). So as the omega-6:omega-3 ratio of the cellular membrane increases in response to the American diet, one becomes more prone to a whole host of diseases, the most common of which is atherosclerotic heart disease. Remember, the vast majority of diseases have an inflammatory component! Why do you think aspirin is an effective combatant of coronary artery disease and cancer? Likely this is due to aspirin's anti-inflammatory actions as opposed to "blood-thinning" effects.

And yet you don't necessarily need medications to reduce bodily inflammation. To prevent heart disease, the number number one killer of Americans, and to potentially reduce the incidence of certain cancers among many other diseases, *one must alter the omega-6:omega-3 ratio!* How? Dietary modifications: decreased omega-6 consumption and increased omega-3 fatty acid consumption. That means NO French fries, as these are essentially *bathed in arachidonic acid* and to add insult to injury, cooked at a high temperature. Increase your consumption of small, cold-water fish (e.g., sardines and mackerel). I'm not a fish eater, yet I take high-dose omega-3 capsules around the clock. For me, it's not an apple but an *oil change* a day that keeps the doctor away.

Why has omega-3 intake come to the forefront recently? Is it because of their newly discovered anti-inflammatory effects? No. Scientists have known about their metabolic benefits for many years. What we *have* come to learn relatively recently is the importance of inflammation in the genesis of age-related disease, diseases which are, to a great degree, environmental in etiology. Yes, we are killing ourselves through excessive consumption of sugar, omega-6 fatty acids relative to omega-3's, and commercially manufactured fat substitutes such as *trans fatty acids* or *trans fats*. Someone famous once said "We have met the enemy and he is us."

No Trans Fats!

Trans fats are chemically modified (hydrogenated) forms of vegetable oil, originally produced (and added to food) to thwart spoiling. Commercial baked goods and many fried foods, such as doughnuts and French fries, may contain trans fats. Margarines and shortenings may also contain significant amounts of trans fats. Aside from adding taste and texture to various foods, they are otherwise toxic to one's body. The consumption of trans fats is associated with decreased testosterone levels and increased incidence of coronary artery disease, Metabolic Syndrome, and type II diabetes. They raise LDL and lower HDL. Another shocker: There is an increased incidence of various cancer types (colon, breast, and prostate) in patients consuming excessive amounts of trans fats. In this light, I offer you some friendly advice: **avoid trans fats (often disguised as *partially hydrogenated oil* on food labels) like the plague**.

Acknowledging the dangers of trans fat consumption, The New York City Board of Health issued a ban on artificial trans fats in restaurant food. Interestingly, this was associated with a substantial and statistically significant decrease in the trans fat content of purchases at fast-food chains, without a commensurate increase in saturated fat. And such bans have been instituted in at least a dozen jurisdictions including the *state* of California! The message is loud and clear.

The Truth about Cholesterol

In stark contrast, a message that has repeatedly fallen on deaf ears concerns cholesterol. Cholesterol has been vilified for years! Elevations in cholesterol, you've been told, place you at a higher risk for heart attack and stroke, right? Likely not. Elevations in oxidized LDL ("bad" cholesterol), particularly subtype B, in an inflammatory milieu, do however increase your risk for a vascular event. I'll say it again: **the oxidative and inflammatory status of the body is a key determinant of one's health**. We are stratified, either susceptible or protected from disease, based on our inflammatory or oxidative burdens.

Cholesterol, in the genesis of atherosclerotic disease, is a **REPARATIVE** molecule that accumulates at sites of injury

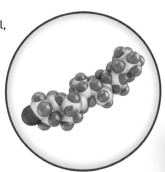
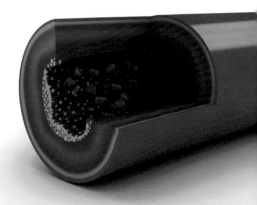

So what is cholesterol and why is it important? Cholesterol is *vital* to our existence, as are fats. This waxy substance is the precursor of many hormones including cortisol, testosterone, progesterone, and estrogen. In fact, it is considered the "mother of all hormones." Cholesterol is also a crucial component of cell membranes, including the myelin sheaths of neurons. Statin drugs (Lipitor, Mevacor, etc.) that inhibit cholesterol synthesis interfere with production of these critical molecules, oftentimes causing more harm than good. Therefore, statins must be used extremely carefully, and only in select patient populations. Unfortunately, due to the aggressive scare tactic-based marketing schemes utilized by Big Pharma, most individuals with "high cholesterol" are prescribed statins. As a *preventive* modality for coronary heart disease. Well guess what? The data don't pan out. A 2010 meta-analysis of more than 65,000 patients (including data from 11 randomized trials) concluded that **the use of statins in a high-risk primary prevention setting was not associated with a statistically significant reduction in the risk of all-cause mortality**. Read that last sentence again. Now go show it to your doctor. *That's* the data. And here's the source:

Ray KK, et al: Statins and all-cause mortality in high-risk primary prevention: a meta-analysis of 11 randomized controlled trials involving 65,229 participants. *Arch Intern Med.* 2010 Jun 28; 170(12):1024-31.

That being said, statins are appropriate in middle-aged men with previous histories of heart disease (PROSPER trial) but the effect is modest.

I introduced the topic of cholesterol in this manner because I purposely wanted to downplay the importance of cholesterol, seen on your yearly lab tests as an absolute number. The majority of cholesterol is synthesized in the liver, while the remainder is taken in from dietary sources. Hepatic synthesis is a function of genetics (this you can thank mom and dad for). In fact, there's no connection whatsoever between cholesterol in food and cholesterol in blood. So stop obsessing over the egg yolk you may have eaten yesterday as it pertains to your "Total Cholesterol" number. Instead, concern yourself with the subtypes of LDL floating around in your blood and your triglyceride:HDL ratio, each of which can be optimized with dietary interventions and not by default with statins.

Cholesterol, in the context of coronary artery disease, is what I would call an "epiphenomenon." In addition to being a hormonal precursor and an integral part of cellular membranes, cholesterol deposits *are* found in coronary artery plaques at the time of bypass surgery. We see them! Does their *presence* vilify them? Are the plaques themselves the culprit, or is something else going on?

Have you ever heard of guilt by association? Doctors call this "true-true-unrelated." A cholesterol plaque is resident within the endothelium: *true*. The patient is undergoing a procedure in which said cholesterol plaques are being "bypassed" to re-establish blood flow: *true*. Logic would dictate that high cholesterol **caused** the plaque formation and, henceforth, the need for the surgery. Umm… No. Unrelated. High cholesterol does not ultimately condemn you to a cardiac or cerebrovascular event, let alone a bypass procedure (70 percent of which are performed for unindicated reasons in the first place).

Cholesterol, in the genesis of atherosclerotic disease, is a reparative molecule that accumulates at sites of injury. It is shuttled around the body and delivered to cells by a carrier, low-density lipoprotein or LDL. There it is used for membrane construction, or for the conversion into other metabolites, such as the steroid hormones. HDL, or high-density lipoprotein, serves an opposing function to that of LDL: to remove cholesterol from cells (and other lipoproteins) and return it to the liver to be excreted in the bile. Its benefit to the cardiovascular system is by reducing the amount of *deposited* cholesterol in the vascular endothelium. *Deposited. In areas of injury.* LDL does not accumulate in the endothelium in a haphazard manner. It does as an adaptive response to a stimulus. As arthritis accumulates in your spine ("spurs") as a means to stabilize an ill-moving joint, so too does LDL accumulate at a site damaged by mechanical stress (hypertension, for example) or toxins such as cigarette smoke. And it is *oxidized* LDL that is atherogenic. Native LDL is never a problem until exposed to thieving free radicals which steal an electron, rendering the LDL particle highly reactive. Remember, oxidative stress and free radical production occur after a high glycemic index-carbohydrate meal. In this inflammatory milieu, native LDL is oxidized, and accumulates at sites of endothelial injury, particularly LDL subtype B. The atherogenic cascade is then initiated, ultimately culminating in potentially vaso-occlusive plaque formation.

So cholesterol, for many years demonized, is not the culprit. Inflammation, free radical formation and associated oxidative stress, and sugar consumption literally are the proverbial 'boys who stole the cookie jar.' Cholesterol, the usual suspect, is merely the bystander as evidenced by the outright failure of myriads of statin trials. Lowering cholesterol pharmacologically is akin to treating an infection with pain medications, as opposed to eradicating the organism with antibiotics. You wouldn't do that, would you? Well, have a look around. Better yet, have a look in your medicine cabinet. For years this has been the trend. "Lower cholestero*l at all costs!*" mandated Big Pharma. And statin sales escalated, despite evidence of their limited utility.

Enter the low-fat diet. These were created under the notion that reduced fat intake equates to reduced cholesterol, and reduced cholesterol to reduced vascular risk. We know the latter to be untrue. And while there may be a reduction in LDL when saturated fat intake is reduced, there is subtype shift from LDL 'A' to 'B', hence an increased coronary risk. In addition, one sacrifices the HDL-bolstering effect of saturated fat intake through so-called low-fat diets. A misnomer, these diets should be renamed "low-fat/more carbohydrate," as fat is often replaced with carbohydrate. This is manifested as elevated triglycerides and reduced HDL cholesterol. Reduced vascular risk from a low fat diet? Not necessarily.

Better Than Low Fat—The Right Balance

A 2011 meta-analysis inclusive of six trials and 2650 patients, compared the efficacy of a Mediterranean (30-40 percent of calories from fat) to a low-fat diet for modifying cardiovascular risk factors. Mediterranean diets appear to be more effective than low-fat diets in inducing clinically relevant long-term changes in cardiovascular risk factors and inflammatory markers. This result was corroborated by a second 2013 study published in the *New England Journal of Medicine*. In a multicenter trial in Spain, 7447 participants at high cardiovascular risk but with no cardiovascular disease at enrollment were randomly assigned to one of three diets: a Mediterranean diet supplemented with extra-virgin olive oil, a Mediterranean diet supplemented with mixed nuts, or a control diet (with advice to *reduce dietary fat*). Those patients on the Mediterranean diet had nearly a **30 percent reduction** in major cardiovascular events (myocardial infarction, stroke, or death from cardiovascular causes) relative to those in the control group.

This study is not suggesting that low-fat diets do not work, mind you. They do work, *provided high-glycemic index carbohydrates do not replace the fats*. The health-promoting effects of the diet also stem from reduced intake of omega-6 fatty acids (which are inflammatory in nature, remember?). In years past, omega-6 intake was encouraged as a substitute for animal fat. Vegetable oils such as corn oil, sunflower, safflower, soybean, and cottonseed oil, as well as margarine were touted by public health authorities as "heart-healthy." However, the data suggests otherwise. An updated meta-analysis, including recovered data from the Sydney Diet Heart Study (a 458-person cohort), demonstrated that substitution of dietary linoleic acid (omega-6) in place of saturated fats increased the rates of death from all causes, coronary heart disease, and cardiovascular disease. So scrap the Crisco and the margarine. Up your intake of omega-3 fatty acids instead! Think not just lower cholesterol at all costs, but *at all costs lower inflammation.*

Do you notice a theme here? **Keeping inflammation in check is paramount to disease prevention.** And an "anti-inflammatory" diet is nothing short of *foundational* in one's quest for health. Daily exercise will not compensate for poor nutrition. In fact, it may further burden the body with free radicals! Your fitness goals will never be realized if you make the wrong food choices; health will be yours, however, if you choose wisely. But as always, *those* choices are yours. You are not a byproduct of your environment, nor the victim of "bad genes." Ultimately, if you have the knowledge, and the *confidence* to make the right choices, health will be yours. Because health begins in the mind. What else would you expect a neurosurgeon to say?
(But it's true...)

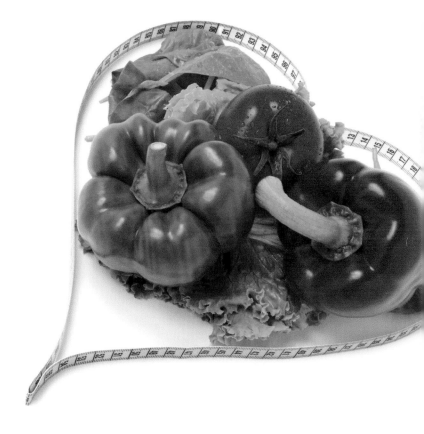

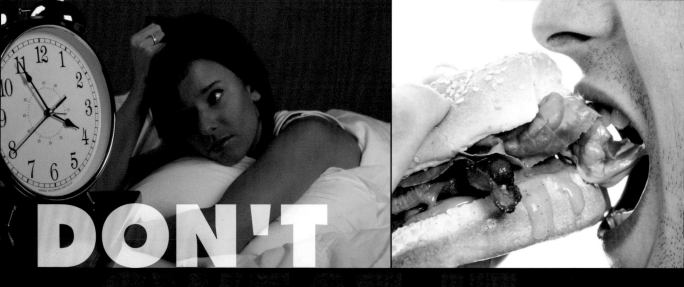

DON'T
SWEAT IT

STRESS ASSUMES MANY FORMS. There is the physical stress associated with exercise, environmental stress derived from pesticides laden food (toxins), and psychological stress often times associated with work, or interpersonal relationships, to name a few. Stress is everywhere; we are continually bombarded with stressors every day of our lives.

But as always, **you have a choice.** Fall victim to its effects and be stricken with disease, or utilize it to better yourself and prevent disease! The beneficial effects of *acute* bodily stress were discussed previously in the chapters on strength training. Now let's talk about the opposite side of the coin, the damaging effects of stress on the body. Poison front-man Brett Michaels put it best, "Every rose has its thorn." Well, in the case of stress, the thorn undoubtedly outsizes the flower.

Just the word "stress" conjures up negative images, doesn't it? It has a bad connotation. And rightfully so. Stress kills, plain and simple. And it takes its toll surreptitiously, flying under the radar like a stealth bomber on a nighttime mission. Lurking and wreaking havoc on

the body with surgical precision. Disastrous. And frightfully intangible. Stress can't be measured directly. There are no specific lab tests for it. Doctors can't order a blood "stress level." We see only the *effects* of its wrath: accelerated aging and predisposition to age-related disease (statistically what is most likely to kill you, remember). Skeptical? See for yourself then. Have a look at the skin or the physique of an avid marathon runner? Aged. Physically aged. Why? Because long distance running stimulates massive free radical release that *decimates* bodily tissue, stealing electrons from vital cellular structures akin to a thief pillaging a bank of its holdings. In addition, the induced sarcopenia (muscle loss) compromises one's immune system. The stronger live

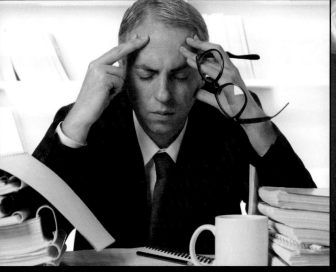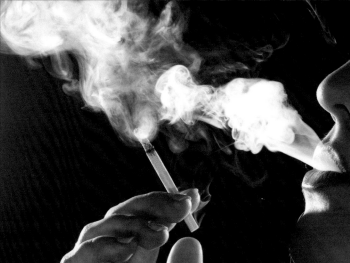

longer, right? Cumulatively, the assumed stresses of chronic long distance running are simply not worth the *assumed* benefits. In my opinion, it's just plain stupid. Strive to minimize stress instead of burdening yourself with more!

Its silent workings make this difficult at times however. The American diet, for example, is laden with pesticides and other carcinogens. That being said, for many of us, *food* itself stresses the body. An environmental stressor like tobacco smoke, foods high in simple carbohydrates wreak havoc on the cardiovascular system, promoting atherosclerotic disease and predisposing one to both heart attack and stroke. Its association with free radical production accelerates aging, and more specifically "inflamm-aging," the process we are desperately trying to slow! Don't add fuel to the proverbial fire. Instead let's use food to fortify ourselves. To quote Hippocrates, "Let food be thy medicine and medicine be thy food." Makes sense, doesn't it? Eating properly will allow us to better adapt to *other* external stressors running rampant in today's society.

Psychological stressors on a chronic basis initiate cascades of hormonal responses (increased cortisol and epineph-rine production) which ultimately serve a destructive, catabolic effect. Have you ever worked a stressful job with a nasty, ever-berating boss? We've all dealt with toxic personalities at some point, right? There was no shortage during my neurosurgery residency, I assure you, and by virtue a lot of imposed stress. Most of us coped, but some faltered under the, at times, "mind-numbing" pressure, and led a miserable seven-year existence (one individual had repeated bouts of diverticulitis, for example). Unchecked, psychological stress can and *will* take its toll, especially as we age. Not only is the brain less resistant to insults (those verbal included), but the body secondarily is as well. Muscle mass declines and chronic blood sugar elevations promote the development of insulin resistance and the **Metabolic Syndrome,** a potential harbinger of disaster. Our immune system is by virtue compromised and disease sets in.

The same occurs with lack of sleep. Insomnia and poor sleep habits, in general, are associated with weight gain, chronic fatigue, and a predisposition to a variety of diseases. Let's face it, your brain performs a much needed "reboot" during sleep. Neurotransmitters we hear about these events? **Often.** No one is immune to the effects of stress, not even you. Running 10 miles a day does *not* compensate for a two-pack-per-day tobacco habit. On the contrary in fact, these multi stressors working synergistically **will kill you!** Having removed many metastatic tumors from patient's brains, I make it really simple for my patients, "You smoke, you die." Harsh? Check the statistics. They're provided to you jokingly as a courtesy of Philip Morris and R.J. Reynolds.

I charge you to keep stress in check. Directly address and eliminate the offending agent(s) or cope with it through meditation or yoga, or even something more basic like reading a book. Take time out of your day to listen to music or take a walk just to clear your head. Play golf or swim off stress. Find a hobby that engages you. Options abound. The method is for *you* to choose! I love riding my motorcycle and waterskiing barefoot with my kids. *My* choices, no one else's. Don't even discuss this with your neighbor, as your needs are likely different from his or hers. Do what is best for *you* to minimize stress. This is intangible, but is extremely critical to your health. Trust me on this, I am living proof. Just consider what I do for a living...

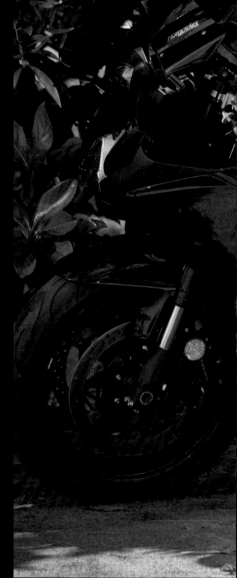

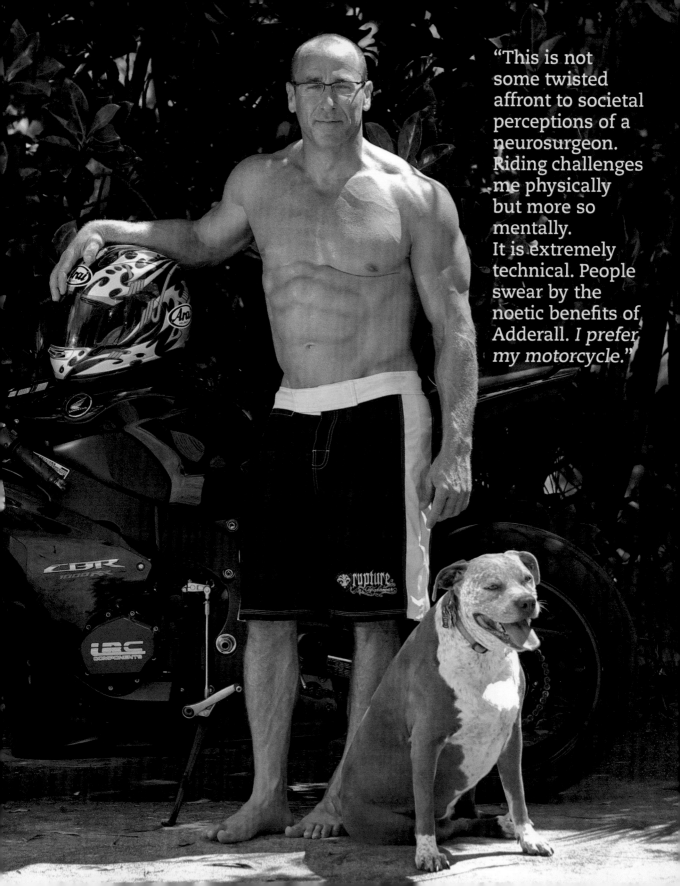

"This is not some twisted affront to societal perceptions of a neurosurgeon. Riding challenges me physically but more so mentally. It is extremely technical. People swear by the noetic benefits of Adderall. *I prefer my motorcycle.*"

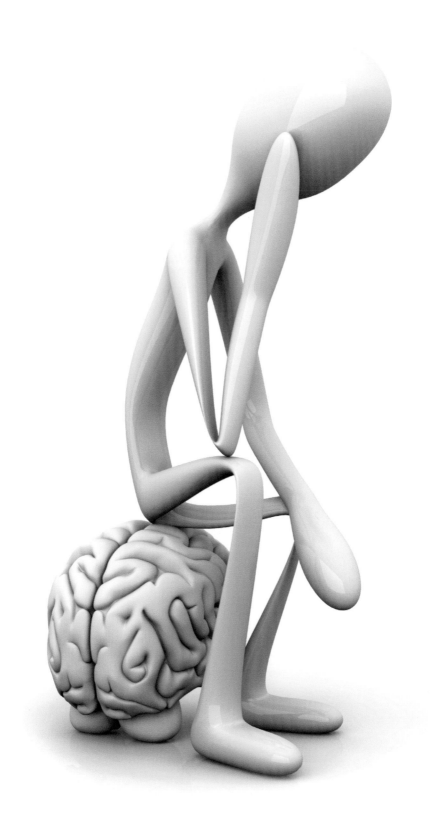

DON'T forget your BRAIN

You saw this one coming! I mean, what credible neurosurgeon would exclude a chapter on the brain? It is THE only organ in the body worth discussing, right?
Of course, I'm kidding...

Although cardio-thoracic surgeons and neurosurgeons jokingly argue about which organ outranks the other, the reality is, you couldn't live without either one of them. The problem is, people take both organs for granted. They neglect them, and at times, abuse them. It's a sad fact that people take better care of objects that can be easily replaced, than they do their own bodies! If you've ever bought a new car, you know what I mean. Remember how careful you were those first few months? You handled it with kid gloves and hyper-vigilance. You parked it in the safest spots where you were least likely to get scraped and you shied away from potholes in the road that could wreck your alignment. You filled it with premium gas. You garaged it to protect it from the elements that can cause it to rust. The thrill wears off, and eventually you get a little less compulsive, but that's ok, because down the road, you know you can replace it.

Now think about the care and attention that you give your brain and your heart. Do you exercise regularly? Are you careful about the "fuel" you feed it? Do you consume enough antioxidants to protect your organs from free radicals that can cause your body to "rust out?" Probably no! And unlike a car, you can't trade in these two vital organs for better models when they start to run down. They are with you for a lifetime. And don't come to this realization after your first heart attack or stroke, after your first bout of crushing chest pain or slurred speech.

I *have* taught you something, right? That **prevention is the best treatment.**

In reality, your brain and your heart are not competing for your attention: what works for one, will help the other. Stroke prevention methods are virtually identical to those for heart attack prevention. After all, they're both vascular diseases. A heart attack and a "brain attack" (stroke) are similar pathophysiologically. Feeder arteries fail to provide adequate blood flow to the heart or brain respectively, the tissue becomes ischemic, and ultimately dies (*and you may, as well*). In the case of the heart, its pumping action falters. That of the brain, a myriad of symptoms may become apparent. Various syndromes may occur, some extremely unsettling. In fact, books have been written about neurological oddities such as "alien hand" syndrome and Gerstmann's syndrome. [One example is *The Man Who Mistook His Wife for a Hat*, authored by neurologist Oliver Sacks. Great read.] My point? The complexity of the brain cannot be overstated. Relative to what we know about the heart for example, and despite massive research efforts, little is known about the brain.

The brain is not a muscle. It is not a blood pump. It is an amorphous mass of interconnected neurons or nerve cells which are primarily insulated by fat. The brain is the most complex object in the known universe, composed of 80-100 billion neurons and *approximately 10 thousand trillion* interconnections. That was not a typo. You have 10 quadrillion neuronal connections between your ears, many of which are organized into complex networks that serve a variety of functions. And most of these we take for granted! Do you have to think in order to follow a passing car traveling down the street? What about catch a baseball? These processes occur almost automatically after being put into motion. How? The brain performs an enormous amount of background processing without it reaching the threshold of awareness, similar to a computer. In fact there are neuronal circuits that modulate our level of *awareness!* Ever seen a boxer or MMA fighter get knocked out? This is due to transient malfunction of this circuitry in contrast to *coma* which heralds more significant dysfunction or frank damage to these critical pathways.

And the brain is packed with such micro-circuitry, some of which may be "accessed" through volition or thought, and some inaccessible. No matter. Every square centimeter of your brain is critical, despite elements of redundancy, plasticity (as we've come to appreciate in recent years) and even so-called "silent areas." It was once thought that we utilize only a small percentage of our brains. B.S. Nearly every brain region is active. By no logical mechanism would a human evolve with a brain 90 percent of which is inactive! It would make no sense. Remember, *natural selection teases out efficiency and eliminates waste*, ever optimizing. Why do you think the brain's surface appears corrugated and in-folded upon itself, for example? To maximize surface area! To pack more neurons into the finite volume of the skull, the operative word being "packed."

Neuronal density of the brain is extremely high. For example, your ability to understand language *or* multiple languages is localized to a region of only 15-20 cm^2, or about the size of a silver dollar. This obviously is "very expensive real estate," as neurosurgeons say when contemplating an operation even remotely close to such *eloquent* brain (no pun intended). Truth be told, with a neuronal density of 50,000 per cubic millimeter of cerebral cortex, *all brain tissue is pricey.* Childhood memories for example could be forever lost from strategic damage to a small region of the brain, stroke-induced damage for example. We've talked book-loads about risk factors for stroke, right? Well think about it. Vascular disease is vascular disease. *And whether the process affects the heart or brain, it's all the same* (the rhyme was unintentional; it is catchy though).

Prevent Heart Attack, Prevent Stroke

Because the brain's neuronal density is so high, it *demands* a significant amount of blood flow. While the brain represents only about 2 percent of your total body mass, it accounts for more than 25 percent of the blood flow. Three quarters of a liter of blood bathe the brain per minute, providing it with necessary oxygen and glucose. How else would those billions of neurons stay alive? Does your laptop's CPU *require* power? Of course it does.

The fact that the brain requires a massive amount of blood makes it susceptible to states of low blood flow. Turn the supply of glucose and oxygen off even for *seconds* and it results in a stroke, which kills off precious neurons. It's exactly the same mechanism as a heart attack, with exactly the same

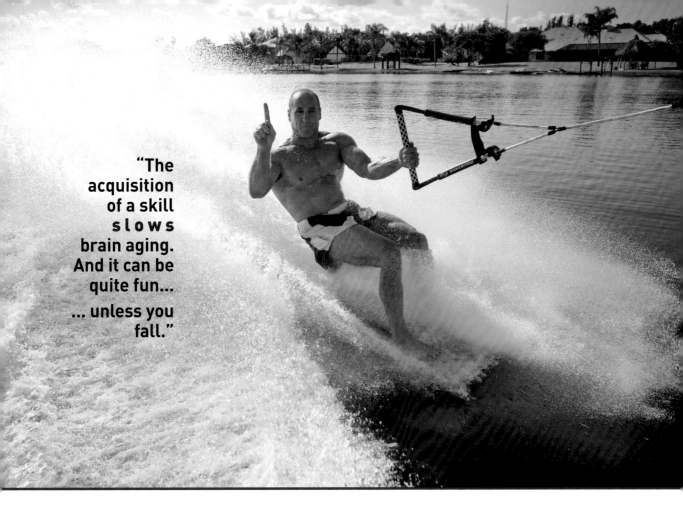

"The
acquisition
of a skill
s l o w s
brain aging.
And it can be
quite fun...
... unless you
fall."

risk factors. Brain attack or heart attack—they're both *vascular* diseases. It shouldn't surprise you, therefore, that patients with coronary artery disease often have significant carotid atherosclerosis as well. The "carotid arteries" are the main pipelines to the brain and are particularly prone to plaque development. So much so, that heart surgeons check the carotid arteries with an ultrasound test *prior* to performing bypass surgery, and if severely diseased, they're cleaned out concomitantly during what is known as an "endarterectomy." Kill two birds with one stone...

Large trials have demonstrated the efficacy of such procedures for stroke prevention. Truth be told, you shouldn't resort to an endarterectomy as a preventive modality. Don't allow yourself to get to that point! Identify risk factors for vascular disease early on and mitigate your risk through diet, supplementation, exercise and stress reduction. We've been through this, many times. My point? By protecting your heart with lifestyle modifications, you are concomitantly protecting your brain and every tissue and cell in your body as well.

Work Your Brain, Protect Your Brain

Exercise is protective of the heart, we all know that. The transient stress imposed on the heart (by the working muscles) makes the heart a more efficient pump through a variety of mechanisms that will not be detailed here. Suffice it to say that getting your heart rate up every day is beneficial. Sitting on your ass all day exerts just the opposite effect.

As detailed elsewhere in this book, your brain benefits from exercise as well. I know, it's not a muscle. Physiologically, mechanistically and structurally, it is in no way related to muscle. But it can be worked as muscle is worked during exercise.

Exercise forges neural pathways in the brain. Let's face it, there is a component of learning in exercise. As you learn to write with your left hand, for example, you learn to properly execute a squat. The process of learning literally rewires the brain. That's why it takes time. You cannot master the squat overnight. Why? The brain has to change. Neuronal connections or "synapses" are formed through very complex biophysical mechanisms under the influence of growth factors such as NGF (nerve growth factor) and BDNF (brain-derived nerve factor).

These "neurotrophins" provide neuroprotection, exert anti-inflammatory effects on the brain, reverse age-associated spatial memory loss, and enhance learning. Akin to foods with high levels of antioxidants, NGF and BDNF act as free radical scavengers as well. And you know what free radicals do to your brain? Let's put it this way: free radical-induced damage has been implicated in the genesis of neurodegenerative diseases such as Parkinson's and Alzheimer's.

In the Alzheimer's brain, there is noted degeneration of "cholinergic" neurons, the subset of neurons which use a chemical known as acetylcholine to talk to one another. These are critical to the formation of new memories which is why grandma can't remember what she had for dinner last night, yet recalls the names of her childhood friends. Tell grandma to get more exercise! Studies have shown that the associated up-regulation of nerve growth factor (NGF) could reverse the destruction of cholinergic neurons seen in the Alzheimer's brain.

But don't wait until you develop Alzheimer's dementia to start running. Start now! *Increased physical activity is protective of the brain as it prevents the progression of age-related brain atrophy.* And this is not only inclusive of the brain's memory centers, but of every region of the brain. Yes, neuronal death is inhibited by physical activity. This too is likely a function of stimulated expression of nerve growth factors. There is also recent evidence that the augmented blood flow to the brain during exercise promotes neurogenesis. Exercise can enhance both your learning abilities and memory!

How else can you turbo-charge your brain? Easy. Learn a new skill (like a properly executed squat or a deadlift). Or what about a new language? Try holding your fork with your non-dominant hand. Can you juggle three balls? No? Well then learn. I routinely do problems from SAT or LSAT prep books under time constraint to keep my mind sharp (in addition to keeping up with my ever-endeavoring children).

Daily mental challenges are important, but not because they will make you "smarter" as is often advertised by those standing to earn millions, effectively selling intelligence. I mean, who doesn't want to be smart? Mental exercise like physical exercise is task specific. As discussed in another chapter, the concept of "functional training" is bunk. You don't swing a weighted golf club to better your swing. This does not work! And may in fact prove detrimental. One task does not translate to the other. The best way to better your golf swing is to… play golf! And the same is true for your brain. It is unlikely that your I.Q. will skyrocket as a result of these "brain games," however you may become a more astute test taker or a more efficient problem solver. And that may provide some collateral benefit. The magnitude of this effect is a topic of ongoing debate in fact. Is it that intelligent adults do crossword puzzles or are the crosswords to some degree making them intelligent?

My 96-year-old grandmother for instance, did crosswords into her final days. Sharp as a tack, she routinely took me to school in the daily word scramble. I was both mortified yet proud at the same time. Was it her voracious appetite for books and the daily Jumble® that fostered intelligence, or was it her intelligence that demanded she read and challenge herself with puzzles? All I know is that she remained "smart" until the very end, which is what we all aspire to.

Smart Drugs

We've all heard about drugs that reportedly make you smart, so-called "smart drugs" or nootropics. But is this myth or reality? I can tell you one thing for sure: many pharmaceuticals are being used as "neuro-enhancers." In Europe, where regulations are less stringent, many brand-name drugs are utilized off-label to enhance cerebral blood flow, increase the concentration of a particular neurotransmitter, and/or stimulate neurogenesis. These include Hydergine, Deprenyl and Prozac (respectively) to name a few. Yes, Prozac (that wasn't a typo) has been shown to enhance neurogenesis in patients who have suffered a stroke. Whether or not this will ultimately translate into a *functional* improvement in healthy individuals is unknown.

There are some smart drugs that are also available over-the-counter: They are sold as nutritional supplements. Below, I review some of my favorites.

PIRACETAM

In my opinion, the oldest and most popular is Piracetam, the mechanism of action of which remains unclear. Its index 1976 study involving college students demonstrated improvements in verbal learning after 14 days. This smart drug has also been shown to have a variety of positive effects in patients with cognitive disorders (i.e. dementia) and epilepsy. The side effect profile of Piracetam, marketed interestingly as *Nootropil*, is very benign; the reported side effects like headache and irritability are mild.

Dosage: 800 mg twice daily.

VINPOCETINE

Derived from the periwinkle plant, vinpocetine is a smart drug that has been demonstrated to have potent anti-inflammatory effects which is at least partly responsible for its beneficial effects on demented patients. Remember, *inflammation* is a key component in the pathogenesis of Alzheimer's disease and other neurodegenerative conditions. Vinpocetine also improves neuronal plasticity, blood flow to the brain and maintains healthy levels of neurotransmitters. It has anti-seizure activity in animal models as well, stabilizing the brain. Available with a prescription in Europe, Vinpocetine was historically used for age-related memory decline. In the context of its reported effects on the brain, we Americans use it as a neuro-enhancer. And you can buy it in most health food stores!

Dosage: 10mg, 1-3 times daily.
Caution: Speak to your doctor before starting Vinpocetine as there may be an interaction between it and blood-thinning medications.

GINGKO BILOBA

Everyone has heard of the next one: ginkgo biloba. I've personally witnessed many people buying ginkgo in the health food store; they've been told "it's good for the brain." And there's likely truth to it. Ginkgo exerts its effects by increasing levels of neurotransmitters in the brain, reducing blood viscosity and quenching free radicals (as an antioxidant). Do you notice a trend here?

Several small studies have substantiated ginkgo's beneficial effects on performance in tests of attention and memory. And while larger randomized trials have yielded inconsistent results, there clearly is promising evidence of improvement in cognition and function associated with ginkgo. Some individuals use prescription drug donepezil (Aricept) in an effort to thwart off Alzheimer's disease. Why not use ginkgo instead? A trial comparing the two in fact demonstrates similar efficacy in the treatment of mild to moderate Alzheimer's disease. So save your money (and your brain). Add ginkgo to your regimen.

Dosage: 100-600 mg daily.
Caution: As ginkgo is a blood thinner, discuss its usage with your doctor.

PREGNENOLONE

Last but not least is pregnenolone. It's literally a steroid hormone for the brain, similar in structure to progesterone. And we know progesterone does wonders for the brain, right? Pregnenolone has come to the forefront recently, possessing numerous potential benefits. As it or its derivatives play roles in myelinization and confer neuroprotection, studies have demonstrated benefit in animal spinal cord injury models and in those designed to assess learning and memory. But are these studies applicable to humans? Large randomized trials simply do not exist.

We do know that pregnenolone is found in high concentrations in the healthy brain. It's made there! Levels fall however as you age, and its neuroprotective effects by virtue, are diminished. Your memory begins to deteriorate. Sometimes depression sets in...

Pregnenolone levels are significantly reduced in the cerebrospinal fluid of depressed patients which bespeaks its potential as a non-pharmaceutical therapeutic. In fact, among users, pregnenolone has often been labeled as the "happiness hormone" on the basis of its mood enhancing effects, but don't assume you have to be depressed to use it!

Dosage: 50 mg daily
Caution: Keep in mind too that pregnenolone is a hormone. That being said, there are potential associated side effects (akin to hormone replacement therapy). At low doses however, pregnenolone is very well tolerated. If you have a hormone sensitive cancer, be sure to discuss its usage with your doctor.

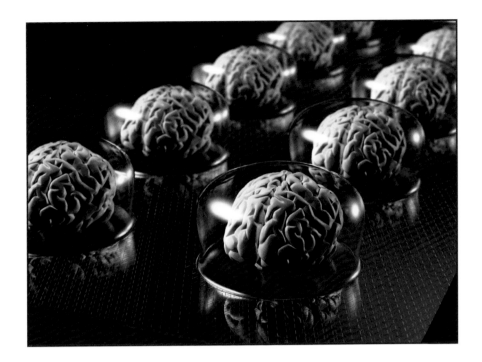

Final Thoughts

You will not become wiser nor become capable of performing differential calculus while speculating on the laws of the universe by virtue of smart drug usage. We simply aren't there yet. In fact, we are only beginning to understand intelligence. I ask you this, what makes someone intelligent, on a neuronal basis? And if we don't know the answer to this fundamental question, how can we augment intelligence? At this point, therefore, it is nothing short of a crap-shoot. Tweak your biochemistry; trial the various smart drugs for three-month intervals at a minimum. Has your work productivity improved? Do you have fewer memory lapses? Is your mood better? Are you having any side effects? Attempt to establish a regimen that suits you best. Or not. At worst, you've spent some hard-earned money. At best, well...

And rest assured, if you choose to pass on the smart drugs yet are taking the 10 recommended supplements detailed later, your brain is fairly well protected. Keep in mind however, that these supplements are part and parcel of a healthy lifestyle, diet and exercise included. *Do not rely on supplements alone to mitigate your risk factors for disease*, be it coronary artery or cerebrovascular disease. They are adjuncts only.

And never forget that these diseases are essentially the same patho-physiologically. Treat one, you treat the other. A healthy body begets a healthy mind. Conversely, a healthy mind begets a healthy body. Of course, I prefer the latter. But don't tell the cardiac surgeons...

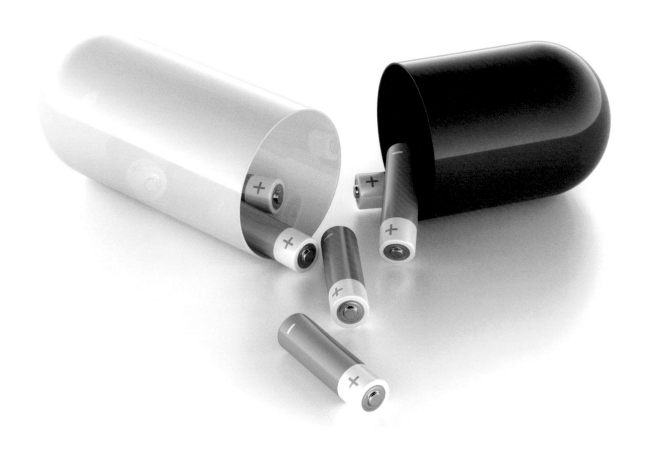

8

SUPPLEMENTS
101

Please consult with your doctor prior to the start of any supplement regimen, as there may be a contraindication that you are unaware of. These drugs have side effects (in my opinion, worth the risk) that must be discussed prior to their initiation. That being said, the medications are typically well tolerated, and I take all of them...

Rarely a day goes by when someone doesn't ask me about what supplements I take to stay in shape. (Note: I am rarely asked about my workout routine or dietary recommendations!) I believe that many people regard supplements as magical elixirs that can fast-track you to a better body.

A case in point is my friend, who I recently encountered while browsing through the supplement shelves in Whole Foods. Karen mentioned that "someone" had told her that "cat's claw" was good for heartburn (GERD), and she wanted my opinion. Karen is severely obese. My first thought was, this woman has much *bigger* battles to fight. What she really needs to do is lose 150 pounds! My guess is, once her weight problem is resolved, her GERD will disappear. I didn't push the subject because I understand that people are very sensitive about their weight, and it wasn't the time or place for me to start prescribing. I did, however, tactfully suggest that she try taking high-dose omega-3 fatty acids, which not only address both her digestive and weight issues to some degree, but I also believe provide the most benefit of any supplement on the market.

There are countless people like Karen, who can't see the forest through the trees. They have little insight into their medical conditions; they lack introspection. Instead of coming to grips with their problem, they look for remedies for ancillary issues. They seek laxative supplements instead of modifying their diets to include at least 20-25 grams of daily fiber and increasing their water intake. They seek supplements touted to lower blood pressure when their diets are laden with sodium and carbohydrate. Obviously, the real and long-lasting solution is to *fix the primary issue first*. The majority of health problems can be solved with dietary modification and daily exercise. (More than 90 percent of chronic diseases are environmental, remember?)

Don't misconstrue this. I am in no way recommending that you abandon nutritional supplements, quite the opposite in fact. I use them aggressively. So should you. But understand their rationale, keeping in mind that they are not cure-alls, but rather *health* "supplements." Supplements are not to be used as primary treatments for ailments that should be otherwise addressed. They are as their name infers, "supplements," to be taken in addition to an optimal diet and lifestyle. They will not, *unto themselves,* remedy your elevated blood sugar, gouty arthritis, and hypertension. Only *you* can. Stop looking for the easy way out (an all too common *ailment* of today's society). I can assure you raspberry ketone, *in isolation*, is not the answer to your obesity. Ignore the sensationalized claims! Dig deep inside yourself prior to stepping foot into the health food store. Forget about cat's claw and cat's foot. Educate yourself, and in the same vein, stop wasting your money.

Big Pharma Enters the Picture

I'm the first to admit that some supplements that are heavily hyped are completely worthless. (You could say the same about many medical procedures and prescription drugs too!) I don't want to beat up on the supplement industry; there are enough people out there doing it. Supplements have been the whipping boys of the health industry since Linus Pauling touted the merits of vitamin C, or before. As they are considered foodstuffs, supplements roam outside the radar range of the FDA. Essentially, anyone can manufacture a supplement; it's as simple as concocting a novel dessert recipe. For better or for worse, this has attracted a significant amount of scrutiny from various governing bodies and their proponents. Quite frankly, Big Pharma is pissed. Supplements, *some of them*, truly have the potential to impact disease incidence and therefore, company revenue. Remember, companies like Pfizer and Merck thrive on the treatment of illness. **There is money in disease, not health.** Due to this, supplement manufacturers have been vilified and touted as the mortal enemy threatening to rob the gravy train. And that's exactly what it is.

The pharmaceutical industry is corrupt. Overtly. Drug trials are falsified. Indications for medications are extended to squeeze every last cent out of patients. Billions, in fact. And yes, supplement manufacturers are similarly culpable with one exception: *there are far fewer deaths associated with such nutrients.* Acetaminophen overdose accounts for an estimated 450 *deaths* each year due to acute liver failure . Tylenol! And what about Vioxx? And Bextra? In 2010, there were 16,451 **unintentional** deaths related to pharmaceutical drugs. Clearly, Big Pharma CEO's didn't receive the "Primum Nil Nocere" memo—(First, do no harm!). Or were they too busy (filling their coffers with gold bars) to read it?

Billions of dollars in pharmaceutical company revenue are potentially lost with widespread acceptance and usage of nutritional supplements. Not surprisingly, there has been backlash in response to this perceived threat. Supplement manufacturers (Life Extension®) have been raided by the FDA, utilizing military-style tactics and dubious studies refuting the efficacy of supplements (when in fact such studies often have serious design flaws). Naysayers abound.

Except, of course, when Big Pharma figures out a way to make money on supplements—then it's a whole different narrative. The efficacy of several key supplements has recently been recognized by the pharmaceutical industry. Ever heard of omega-3 fatty acids or fish oil? What about resveratrol? Of course you have. GlaxoSmithKline invested $1.65 **billion** to purchase Reliant Pharmaceuticals specifically to acquire the manufacturing rights of Lovaza®, an *omega-3* fatty acid supplement that had been vetted by the FDA, therefore classifying it as a pharmaceutical. Yes, you need a prescription for it. And yes, it is expensive as hell: $265.00 per month vs. $35.00 for an OTC substitute! Because it is "pharmaceutical grade." Umm... who cares? Bottom line: the stuff works! For years, claims touting the efficacy of omega-3 fatty acids (in the context of a variety of disease states) have fallen on deaf ears. Until relatively recently. Interestingly, when Big Pharma jumped aboard the bandwagon, so did some of my colleagues. I remember banging my head against the wall in frustration, as I tried to convince a local neurologist of the merits of omega-3 fatty acids. For years this banter continued. Ultimately I threw in the towel, only to find out that she *now* prescribes omega-3 fatty acids to *all* of her patients with memory disorders. Ironically, she'll never *remember* arguing with me. At least we're getting somewhere though, right? Big Pharma steps in, people listen. Right or wrong (and often duped), people listen. Hopefully, the same thing will happen in the case of this next *supplement,* soon-to-turn drug.

Resveratrol is an antioxidant and anti-inflammatory agent found in the skin of red grapes and in the Japanese knotwood plant. It is the molecule suspected to give red wine its cardio-protective effects and may extend *human* lifespan, as it does in experimental animals. GlaxoSmithKline (again) paid a boatload of money for Cambridge-based Sirtris Pharmaceuticals, a biotechnology company synthesizing a proprietary formulation of the compound resveratrol. A *patentable* version of the readily available OTC supplement. In regular English, that means DRUG! Sounds enticing, right? I can just picture the commercials detailing this novel "life extending" drug. Now imagine the riots in doctor's waiting rooms as patients await their prescription for this propagandized, chemically-modified supplement. Who doesn't want to be younger? But akin to Lovaza and the readily available supermarket grade omega-3 fatty acids, this uber-drug will be chemically and functionally similar to the native compound available at Walmart for a quarter of the price. If anything, the guerilla-style marketing tactics employed by the pharmaceutical companies to advertise such drugs will raise awareness of the many benefits of resveratrol. If it's not a household name by now, it will be, and on their dollar no less.

I would urge you not to wait for the launch of this "miracle" drug. GSK has recently internalized Sirtis Pharmaceuticals but continues to research the compound's effect on human metabolism. And unless the drug is fast-tracked through the FDA, years will pass prior to its release. Worry not, it is readily available. But wait, where's the data? My friends, if you are waiting for "the data" that *establishes* the health benefits of nutritional supplements prior to investing your money, you'll be long dead before that "data" is published. The *proof* is in the biochemistry. I again point you to the French Paradox. Research it for yourself. And look at the Japanese. They live on average five years longer than Americans. Seems like they have a secret "anti-aging" strategy, right? Wrong. It's simply high omega-3 fatty acid intake, limited non-vegetable carbohydrates, and daily exercise. The upshot? High insulin sensitivity. And the ingestion of resveratrol has similar effects. It is likely then that resveratrol *will* extend human life. Don't wait for FDA "approval." Its only motivation is money. And **there is money in disease, not health**. So act now! Optimize your diet, exercise, and take the *proper* supplements.

So which ones qualify as "proper?" Well, that's purely a matter of opinion. Everyone is distinct physiologically. Some may be better served with one versus the other ultimately. At this point, however, detailed metabolic testing can be cost prohibitive and therefore not readily available to the masses. I choose to take those supplements that *logically* appear to have the most benefit given the limited available data.

I know what you're thinking. Dr. Osborn is taking excessive amounts of supplements when he is probably getting the necessary amounts of these micronutrients from his food. Wrong. Neither you nor I are obtaining adequate micronutrients from the food we eat. There are two reasons for this truism. One, your diet simply does not provide adequate amounts of cold water fish, green tea, curcumin (in curry powder) and resveratrol to name a few. It doesn't. And two, if you think it does, you're wrong. Our food is nutritionally depleted of vital nutrients, and it is laden with toxins (i.e. pesticides). So don't be fooled by package labeling: *err on the side of supplementing.*

I know what you're thinking. If you take high doses of certain vitamins, you will either "overdose" on them, or your body will dispose of them in what critics of supplements so disparagingly dismiss as "expensive urine." First, the safety profiles of the recommended supplements (and supplements in general) are excellent (far better than that of pharmaceuticals). You are extremely unlikely to overdose. In fact, I have never even heard of a supplement overdose (this does not include ergogenic aids which are often abused). My point? If you can afford to supplement, and your diet and exercise regimens have been optimized, do it! Err on the side of "expensive urine," particularly in regards to vitamin C, as it has been shown to reduce the risk of bladder cancer (yes, that vitamin C sitting in your bladder is a chemopreventive agent!)

So how, from the literally thousands of supplements on the market, do I select the few that I should take? I chose my supplements logically, based upon what we know to be the agents of the aging process and particularly age-related disease. And they are the same: **free radical damage, oxidative stress, and chronic inflammation**. While these to some degree are by-products of *normal* metabolic processes, our systems are easily overloaded despite fairly robust defense mechanisms (antioxidant systems, for example). Therefore, supplementation for most of the non-genetically-endowed populace is essential for health. Listen to me. No, look at the pictures! I am healthier than I've ever been at age 43. My mind is sharp and I'm in better shape than I was as an adolescent. And you can be too! If *you* assume control. To a great degree, you can thwart the development of age-related bodily changes, the accumulation of which leads to disease.

Dr. Osborn's Top Ten Nutritional Supplements

OMEGA-3 FATTY ACIDS

Omega-3 fatty acids: if you could choose one, this would be it! It is by far the best supplement out there for all-around health benefit. There are literally volumes of data demonstrating the beneficial effects of omega-3's stemming from their robust anti-inflammatory and antioxidant capacities. An integral part of your cell membranes (walls surrounding your cells), omega-3 FA (fatty acids) are vital to your health and particularly beneficial to your heart and brain. *You truly are what you eat.*

All fish oil is not created equal. *Do not* buy the first "fish oil" supplement you come across. In fact, stay clear of such supplements, as most are laden with omega-6 FA. And while these fatty acids are needed to mount an inflammatory response (immune system response, wound healing, and muscle repair), I can assure you that your diet supplies *surplus* amounts. Remember the omega-6:omega-3 ratio of the American diet is 20:1; **optimal is 1:1** (Japan is closest with 4:1). Instead, purchase purified omega-3 FA capsules. Pay particular attention to the quantity of omega-3 per capsule and dose accordingly. In the event that you are unable to find purified preparations and have to buy "fish oil," attempt to find those capsules that have the most omega-3 FA per capsule and the least omega-6. *Your goal is to minimize intake of omega-6 FA and maximize omega-3 FA intake.* Do not assume that your "Fish oil 1200" has 1200 mg of omega-3 fatty acids per capsule. It doesn't. Likely it has 300 mg. So don't be fooled! *Read your labels carefully, twice.*

Daily Dosage: In order to optimize that critical omega-6:omega-3 ratio (discussed previously), take this supplement liberally. I recommend a minimum of *3 grams (3,000 mg) daily* in divided doses. Many individuals take 10 to 15 grams daily without adverse effects (Eskimos eat a lot of fish, right?).

Caution: Omega-3 fatty acids may interfere with blood clotting particularly at high dosages (> 3,000 mg daily). Please discuss usage with your doctor particularly if you are taking blood thinners (warfarin) or medications that interfere with platelet function (aspirin, for example). Accordingly, alert your surgeon if you have a procedure scheduled.

Those with allergies to fish should use precautions when taking omega-3 FA. Discuss this with your doctor (and preferably an allergist) *prior to* starting the supplements.

And here's a trick. Bloating, belching, and diarrhea are common side effects of omega-3 supplements. Simply store your capsules in the freezer; the fatty acids will be released in a more delayed manner and these side effects diminished. This may not be a bad idea anyway as it slows down the oxidation process (fish oil can be oxidized prior to its consumption).

RESVERATROL

Discussed previously, resveratrol is one of the compounds found in wine thought to confer protection against coronary events in people consuming a high-fat diet. Remember the French Paradox? There are numerous animal studies demonstrating its life-extending effects. And the biochemistry has, to a great degree, been elucidated. In addition to providing robust anti-inflammatory effects, resveratrol influences the expression of several gene products which influence metabolism.

In past chapters, I've talked about the inflammatory effects of insulin, particularly excess insulin. *Remember, the more circulating insulin, the more bodily inflammation, resulting in more* **inflamm-aging**. People suffering from type II diabetes are ravished by the effects of elevated circulating insulin. They are the poster children for accelerated aging (particularly those who are poorly controlled). Hmm… so what happens when we attenuate the insulin signal? The opposite occurs theoretically: we age slower. And this is precisely the line of logic utilized by those practicing caloric restriction or CR. By no means is this an easy protocol (30 percent reduction in caloric intake); it is not for the faint-hearted. Yet it *potentially* offers life-extending benefits (studies are obviously difficult to perform given the endpoint: *death*). Don't worry! You can derive similar benefits from resveratrol supplementation. Mark my words, a chemical modification of resveratrol *will* be launched one day as an "anti-aging drug." Diabetics, this is an extremely important supplement for you.

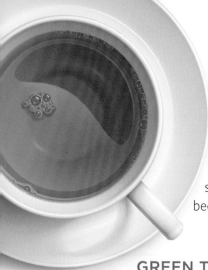

Daily Dosage: *20 mg daily*. For the record, 20-mg resveratrol supplements provide approximately 220 times the amount of resveratrol found in *one* fluid ounce of that red wine the French are drinking! Is it really better to consume more? Would we derive similar benefits from a smaller dose? We simply do not know as longitudinal studies in humans have not been performed.

GREEN TEA EXTRACT

Likely a factor in the enhanced longevity of the Japanese, green tea is a robust antioxidant that has anti-cancer effects probably through its epigallo-catechingallate or EGCG content. EGCG works by protecting cells from lipid peroxidation and DNA damage thought to be integral to atherogenic and neurodegenerative processes. Yes, green tea may slow the progression of Alzheimer's disease by inhibiting plaque formation. Its anti-cancer effects are due to inhibition of tumor angiogenesis (tumor blood vessel formation) and its ability to induce apoptosis (programmed cell death) in tumor cells.

Daily Dosage: *Take a minimum of 900 mg daily* in divided doses. Ideally, one should *drink* several cups of green tea daily if possible (and in this case, scrap the extract).

VITAMIN D$_3$

You may not realize it, but Vitamin D$_3$ is actually a hormone. That's right, it's a vital bodily hormone acting directly on the genome. Once thought to be solely important for bone health and calcium regulation, vitamin D$_3$ has a multitude of additional functions. It likely confers protection against a variety of cancers, is integral to our immune response, has anti-inflammatory properties, influences skeletal muscle growth, and maintains vascular health.

Sadly, the importance of vitamin D$_3$ has gone unrecognized until relatively recently, likely resulting in many needless deaths. In doubt? Here's proof. A large *prospective* study including 18,225 men free of diagnosed cardiovascular disease assessed whether plasma vitamin D$_3$ concentrations are associated with risk of coronary heart disease over a 10-year period. After adjustment for family history of myocardial infarction, body mass index, alcohol consumption, physical activity, history of diabetes mellitus, hypertension, ethnicity, region, marine omega-3 intake, LDL and HDL cholesterol levels, and triglyceride levels, *the relative risk of nonfatal myocardial infarction or fatal coronary heart disease was more than double in those individuals with low vitamin D_3 levels relative to those with normal levels.* **Considering the high prevalence of vitamin D_3 deficiency in the United States, normalization of serum levels would result in more than 100,000 lives saved yearly.** And this only reflects the reduction in fatal *coronary* events. What about cancer-related deaths? You see my point. Take your vitamin D_3! Do not assume for a second that you get adequate sun exposure. You don't. Society is spending more time indoors, as Wii Tennis replaces outings on the clay court. Sunscreen too, while reducing skin cancer risk, can interfere with vitamin D production in the skin.

Daily Dosage: *1,000 -10,000 I.U. daily.* Ask your doctor to check your vitamin D_3 level (a simple blood test). Tailor your daily dosage to attain a level of 50-65 ng/mL.

CURCUMIN

It is suspected that the incidence of Alzheimer's disease in India is approximately **50 percent lower** than that in the United States because of the high quantities of turmeric consumed, a main ingredient of curry powder. Fifty percent! Curcumin (a derivative of the turmeric spice) has powerful antioxidant and anti-inflammatory properties, both of which thwart the formation of amyloid plaque. With regard to the latter, curcumin has been utilized to treat osteoarthritis and inflammatory bowel disease. Researchers are now pursuing its potential anti-cancer (chemopreventive) effects.

Here's the issue. The bioavailability of curcumin is low (i.e. it is poorly absorbed) at oral doses < 4 grams. To remedy this, choose a curcumin preparation with piperine (a black pepper derivative), which has been demonstrated to enhance bioavailability in the first several hours after ingestion. Taking your curcumin with a fish oil supplement may also increase bioavailability by promoting absorption.

Daily Dosage: *800-1,000 mg.*
Caution: Curcumin may interfere with platelet function and therefore blood clotting. Please discuss usage with your doctor particularly if you are taking blood thinners (warfarin) or other medications that interfere with platelet function (aspirin, for example). Alert your surgeon *preoperatively* as well!

B-COMPLEX

These days, you always hear about B-complex vitamins in the context of energy drinks (sheer nonsense!). B-complex vitamins are important for what is termed "methylation," a cellular process that occurs a billion times per second. It's a complicated process involving the transfer of a "methyl" group from one molecule to another. It is critical to the regulation of protein function and gene expression, without which, well, we'd all be goners. Deficient or "hypo" methylation is associated with a variety of diseases such as cancer, coronary artery and cerebrovascular disease, and neural tube defects to name a few. Faulty methylation is associated with elevated homocysteine levels in the blood (more on this later). This often can be remedied by supplementing with B vitamins ("complexed" to include the eight chemically distinct forms). I typically stick with the preparations that have the most folic acid per tablet (with a little bit of searching you will find those with 400 mcg).

Daily Dosage: *1 tablet daily.* And *when*, not *if*, your urine turns bright yellow and quite frankly "stinks," do not equate this to inefficacy or malabsorption of the product. The former is an effect of riboflavin (the Latin word "flavus" means yellow or golden) and the latter, pyridoxine in the preparation.

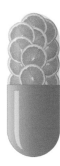

VITAMIN C

Nobel prize winner Linus Pauling alerted us to the vast role that vitamin C plays in the human body. It is integral to numerous biological processes such as tissue repair, the quenching of free radicals (antioxidant), and the formation along with the maintenance of skin, tendons, ligaments, and blood vessels. With regard to the latter, Pauling asserted that chronically low levels of vitamin C ("chronic scurvy") are a cause of atherosclerosis. In the same vein, it has been postulated that a bear's ability to *thwart off* atherosclerotic disease (despite elevated inflammatory markers and high cholesterol levels during prolonged periods of hibernation) is causally related to their *high circulating levels of vitamin C*. Why? Because they synthesize it! And guess what? Humans don't. We must obtain it from our diet or through supplementation. Do not neglect your vitamin C. It is protective of your cells and particularly your vascular endothelium. Statistically, you are likely to die of vascular disease, right? So get a jump on it.

Daily Dosage: *2-5 grams.* Those of you who smoke, err on the high end of that range. Better yet, scrap the cigarettes **now**. Don't be an idiot.

VITAMIN E (mixed tocopherols and tocotrienols)

Firstly, vitamin E does not *cause* prostate cancer, as a recent study suggested. I'm calling bullshit on this one too (as is every respectable scientist vaguely familiar with the flawed study). The poorly designed SELECT study published in *JAMA* utilized 400 IU/day of **all rac-α-tocopheryl acetate,** instead of a *complete* vitamin E supplement, with mixed tocopherols and tocotrienols. This better emulates the vitamin E found in fruits and vegetables. Do fruits and vegetables cause prostate cancer?

The benefits of vitamin E are numerous. For example, supplementation has been demonstrated to reduce atherosclerotic plaque burden and improve one's lipid profile in the context of *complete* preparations. **You will not derive the benefits with α-tocopherol alone**. In fact, α–tocopherol, given in isolation, which is standard for commercial vitamin E preparations, reduces γ–tocopherol levels by 30-50 percent. And guess which one is the far more powerful antioxidant? γ–tocopherol! Do you now see why the SELECT study is ridiculous? The results are spurious. This also highlights the importance of a *complete* vitamin E supplement from which you will derive a variety of protective effects.

Daily Dosage: Select a preparation of *mixed* tocopherols and tocotrienols. I would shoot for one that has a minimum of ***250 mg*** in total of these eight vitamin E components (Vitamin E historically has been α–tocopherol only).
Caution: Vitamin E may interfere with platelet function and therefore blood clotting. Please discuss usage with your doctor particularly if you are taking blood thinners (warfarin) or other medications that interfere with platelet function (aspirin, for example). Alert your surgeon pre-operatively as well. Prior to brain operations, my patients are advised to stop both fish oil and vitamin E supplements (it is extremely rare that I find an individual on curcumin).

MAGNESIUM

Ok, there is no arguing about this one: magnesium stabilizes the heart muscle and prevents arrhythmias. It lowers blood pressure by relaxing blood vessels, plays a role in carbohydrate metabolism and reduces one's risk of osteoporosis by augmenting bone density. And what caliber neurosurgeon would exclude exciting new data on magnesium's effects on the brain? A recently published study suggested that elevation of brain magnesium exerts substantial protective effects in a mouse model of Alzheimer's disease. Specifically, magnesium-L-threonate conferred protection against plaque formation and synaptic (neuron-neuron connection) loss, characteristic of Alzheimer's disease. And this may have treatment implications for humans. 68 percent of Americans are deficient according to a government-sponsored study.

Daily Dosage: *1,000 mg*. Take your magnesium supplement at night, preferably before bed; it will help you sleep.

PROBIOTICS

This is the good bacteria that most of us lack in our gut. Yes, there are "good" bacteria that maintain the health of our bowels, the interface between our bodies and the outside world. Unfortunately, our guts are often overpopulated with "bad" bacteria which interfere with normal physiologic processes, leading to illness. Case in point is antibiotic-associated colitis or "c diff" due to overgrowth of the pathogenic bacteria clostridium difficile. Antibiotics eradicate the *protective* bacteria of the gut. The "bad" bacteria seize the opportunity to multiply, evoking an inflammatory response which can prove fatal (20,000-30,000 Americans succumb *annually* to c. difficile colitis).

There is a very complex bacterial microcosm in one's gut composed of trillions of bacteria. The interactions between the bacteria and the lining of the bowel modulate, via chemical messengers, our immune response and various metabolic processes, which in part dictate insulin sensitivity. Alterations in gut integrity for these reasons can prove disastrous. Unfortunately, this has been underappreciated until relatively recently. If the gut is inflamed, *you* are inflamed. Just because the bowel in actuality is external to the body, does not permit you to neglect it. Nurture it instead for optimal health. Try eating yogurt daily for a week. You'll feel better, guaranteed!

Daily Dosage: (for those not in favor of yogurt) Buy a preparation with *at least 2 billion CFU* (bacteria essentially) per serving. Take one to two servings daily. Double your daily dosage while on antibiotics, or for five days pre-and post-operatively in the event you are having surgery. Another tip: always store your probiotics in the refrigerator. These are live cultures. Would you leave your yogurt out of the fridge for days on end? I think not.

Multivitamin or Not?

Several of the above may be found in multivitamin preparations. In that vein, choose a multivitamin that is just that, "multi," *multiple* capsules or tablets per day. I personally steer clear of the single tablet preparations for two reasons:

1. *The dosages of the individual components are fairly low.* Vitamin C quantities, for example, position one just over the threshold of scurvy. Multi-tablet preps typically contain higher quantities of the micronutrients. My preference is Life Extension® Mix tablets (9 pills daily).

2. *Serum levels of the micronutrients are inconsistent throughout the day.* A steady supply of micronutrients (theoretically provided by a multi-tablet prep) increases the probability of your cells being saturated with vital cofactors around the clock.

Water: An Unsung Hero

While **water** is not considered a supplement, it should be. The majority of people are dehydrated, plain and simple. You may not think you are, but you are. Yes, you! Do you drink 10-12 cups of water daily? Doubtful. Well, this is your water requirement under normal conditions; in extreme conditions, it can be double that amount. Even mild dehydration can affect mental and physical performance. Gastrointestinal function may also be impaired, resulting in delayed transit times and constipation. And while the latter may be unpleasant, even more unpleasant is your prolonged exposure to potential carcinogens as their passage through the gut is delayed. A common cause of constipation is dehydration.

Optimal hydration is associated with a reduced incidence of fatal coronary artery disease, stroke, hypertension, diabetes-related complications such as ketoacidosis, kidney stones and urinary tract infections. Those bouts of dizziness you experience when standing up too abruptly? That may be a function of dehydration. Hydration also affects the fullness of your skin and more importantly its integrity and efficacy as a barrier to pathogens. Remember, you are 60 percent water! It is absolutely essential to life and therefore not to be neglected, although often is.

So "supplement" aggressively with water, *1 gallon per day* as a rule (unless instructed otherwise by your doctor), bodyweight aside. Your urine should be clear and odorless. That is, unless you just took your B-vitamins...

The "Supplements" You Never Hear About

As usual, there's more here than meets the eye. *Many* pharmaceuticals have off label usages with demonstrable benefit, but are simply not offered to patients. Why? Because they are "off label," and doctors are quite frankly nervous. Of lawsuits. And that's a crying shame. Why? *Because your doctor may be taking them!* In that regard, I have listed several that I consider crucial to health. But first allow me to refresh your memory. What are the two biggest killers *worldwide*? Ischemic heart disease and cerebrovascular disease. Keep that in mind...

ASPIRIN

Long thought of for its anti-platelet (blood thinning) effects, aspirin has anti-inflammatory properties to which its benefits can also be attributed. Remember, *virtually every disease has an inflammatory component to it*. If you tamp down inflammation, it will have an impact on disease incidence and severity. Yes, aspirin even reduces the incidence of a variety of cancers! Its health-promoting effects extend beyond the vascular system, beyond heart attack and stroke. According to a study published recently in *Lancet Oncology*, regular aspirin use reduces the risk of colorectal, esophageal, gastric, biliary, and breast cancer. And by nearly **40 percent.** Good ol' aspirin. Bang for the buck, the best medication there is! As of this writing, 125 tablets of Ecotrin 325 mg cost $7.00, or less than six cents per dose. Its effects are wide-reaching. I would recommend it to everyone age 35 and older, barring any contraindications (i.e. bleeding disorder or active peptic ulcer disease). Don't wait until you're 50 when risk factors for disease have already accumulated (there is evidence that risk factors begin accumulating during adolescence, in fact). So how much should people take? My standard advice is an enteric coated baby aspirin every other day (as a starting dosage).

BETA-BLOCKER AND/OR ACE INHIBITOR

Ever hear of the Framingham Study? Allow me to explain. The Framingham Study investigators followed thousands of men and women over several decades and found an increasing relation between systolic blood pressure, and all-cause cardiovascular mortality. While this relationship is not strictly linear, it goes without saying that hypertension, chronic hypertension in particular, is a key promoter of the atherogenic process. Plaque formation begins with injury to the arterial wall as a result of the increased shear force placed upon it. The response *to the injury* is atherogenesis with progressive arterial narrowing. Your goal: minimize arterial injury. How? Normalize your blood pressure. And then normalize it further. Aim for the *low* end of the "normal" range for your age. Ideally, this should be attained through diet and exercise. Even still, a low-dose antihypertensive may prove beneficial long-term. Both ACE inhibitors and beta-blockers have their merits (and demerits). Discuss these with your physician. And don't be satisfied with serial blood pressures at the high end of the "normal" range for your age group; shoot for a more optimal blood pressure. Treat early and aggressively. *Hypertension is a silent killer.*

STATINS

As most of you probably know, statin drugs can lower cholesterol levels, but what you may not know is how many doctors (like me) are taking these drugs, even those who don't have cholesterol problems. Why? Statins are also potent anti-inflammatory agents. And we all know by now, (it's like beating a dead horse) that chronic inflammation underpins nearly every disease, especially those that kill us! From that standpoint alone, everyone should at least consider discussing statin usage with his or her doctor. Of course this may be contraindicated in the context of a normal lipid profile. Which brings me to my next point.

In previous chapters I had discussed cholesterol, and in particular, why we need it floating around our bodies. Cholesterol is not "bad," yet has been vilified by the pharmaceutical industry, specifically by those companies manufacturing (and profiting from) statins. It is in their best interest to demonize cholesterol, and then present a "miraculous" cure for the masses. As it turns out, for a variety of reasons, statins are not the panacea they've been touted to be *clinically* (when analyzing outcome data). But they *do* aggressively lower cholesterol by inhibiting the rate limiting step in cholesterol synthesis. Therefore, for those at high risk of a coronary event in the context of dyslipidemia, statins are an integral part of treatment. In other cases however, the indications become a bit more fuzzy. Statins have side effects which must be taken into consideration. Myalgias (muscle aches), memory loss, drug-induced hepatitis and statin-associated neuropathies are well described in the literature. So your decision to use statins should not be taken lightly.

I use statins to maintain my LDL 100-110 mg/dL, *no less,* and to drive my CRP (serum inflammatory marker) down to nearly zero. Remember, we rely on cholesterol for endothelial repair and equally as important, for hormone production. And we certainly don't want to interfere with those processes! An ideal lipid profile often times can be obtained with rigorous attention to diet and exercise. Some of us, however, have difficulties reaching the "target" LDL level, as cholesterol production is predominantly a function of our genes, and less so diet, as was once suspected. To me, that equates to more *potentially* oxidized LDL substrate or atherogenic LDL. Remember, native LDL unto itself is harmless (particularly the pattern A subtype); it is the *oxidized* LDL particle which causes the problems. Therefore, keeping oxidative stress in check is more important than your "cholesterol number." As we are burdened by, and in fact, bombarded with oxidative stress on a daily basis, one's antioxidant systems may be overwhelmed (hence the *need* for supplements) and LDL particles oxidized. I choose to utilize statins with the intention of lowering my LDL to "target" levels and increasing my HDL (although quite frankly, niacin, a B-vitamin sold over the counter for a lot less, does a way better job with the latter). The choice is yours. Discuss it with your doctor in light of *your* past medical and family history.

In the event that you choose to take a statin, you **must** supplement with CoQ-10 (available over the counter), as this will reduce the incidence of muscle-related side-effects (pain and dysfunction). You probably know someone who, after being placed on statins, developed leg pain and appropriately stopped the medication. Likely, their physician did not recommend CoQ-10, as many are unaware of this potentially protective agent. Take 200 mg (of CoQ-10) daily should you choose to use a statin; don't even start the statin otherwise.

METFORMIN

Wait, the diabetic drug? You got it. Remember resveratrol? Well guess what, metformin (generic Glucophage) acts on similar enzymatic pathways, increasing insulin sensitivity, and by virtue, reducing the insulin signal. You're probably thinking, "I thought I needed insulin?" You do! But not in excess. This is our nation's biggest risk factor for disease. EXCESS INSULIN. Yes, we need insulin for growth and repair, but *excess* insulin is associated with type II diabetes, atherosclerotic disease, cancer, Alzheimer's disease and hypertension. Need I say more? OK. Reducing the insulin signal secondarily reduces inflammation in animal models; this likely occurs in humans as well, given the *anti-tumoral effects metformin has on a variety of cancers*. This effect too is the result of reduced growth factor expression in response to metformin. It acts at the level of the gene! And its actions are not limited to the insulin signaling pathway; they are wide-reaching, affecting and modulating many bodily processes. As you've heard me say before (in the context of resveratrol), an analog of metformin will one day be launched as an "anti-aging" drug. Why? It mimics the effect of caloric restriction (CR). This significantly extends life in animal models. By reducing the insulin signal and therefore the risk of cancer, diabetes, vascular disease and obesity, it will likely have similar effects in humans. Are you going to wait and see *if* it extends life *prior* to discussing this option with your doctor? Or do you plan to assess the available data and make an educated decision, potentially extending your life? I've been on metformin for years. Not a single untoward effect (although they are reported, albeit infrequently). And no, it typically does not make one hypoglycemic.

Starting Dosage: *500 mg twice daily.* Should you choose to take metformin, you must supplement with additional B vitamins, particularly B12 and folate (which you *should* be on an anyway, right?).

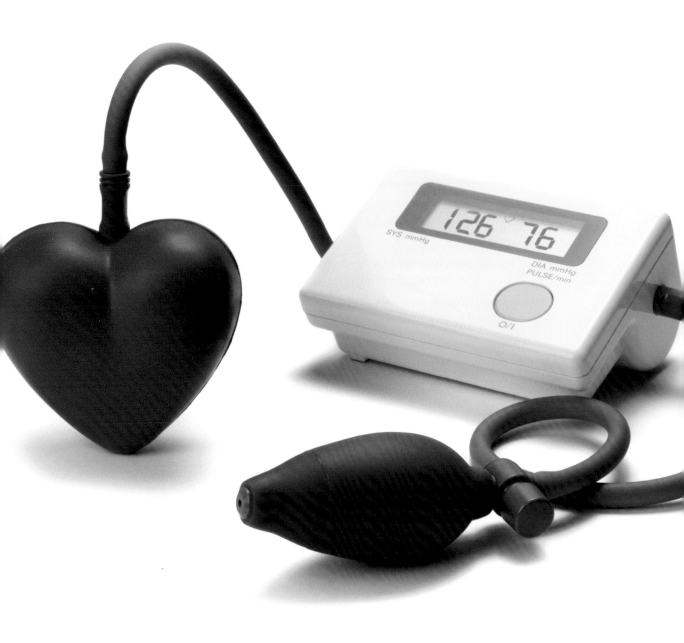

9 Keeping Track:
AT-HOME
MONITORING

Which two diseases kill the most people *worldwide*? Heart attack and stroke. Hands down, these are the two biggest culprits according to the CDC. I know that I've told you this before. If I sound redundant, it's because there's too much at stake here not to make sure that my message is getting through. These two killers are not inevitable. They don't have to happen to you. To a great degree, these diseases can be prevented, or at the very least, their progress slowed.

Keep in mind that *the best treatment for disease is* **prevention**. To prevent disease, however, we must be able to identify risk factors for disease. And yes, there are non-modifiable genetic factors at hand—when it comes to genetic risk factors, some people are dealt a bad hand. What's shocking is that *globally* we can't even control two of the biggest—and preventable—risk factors for vascular disease in general: insulin resistance (prediabetes) and hypertension (high blood pressure) which I discuss in detail below. Why? One reason is that these two often fly under the radar for long periods of time prior to their being discovered. Hypertension and insulin resistance are silent killers, remember. They can do their damage quietly and insidiously, long before someone experiences any symptoms. It is not uncommon for a patient to show up in the ER with previously undiagnosed hypertension and a large hemorrhage in the brain. Or from a heart attack, or in a coma from previously undiagnosed diabetes.

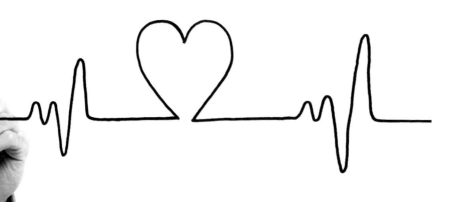

Another related reason is that in general, surveillance is poor. We simply are not aggressive enough. Have you asked yourself the question, "What risk factors for disease do I have?" No? Not good. Don't for one second think that your doctor is going to be able to discover all your risk factors and save you in the nick of time. More often than not, that doesn't happen. The bottom line: *you have to assume responsibility for your own health.*

Given the prevalence of both high blood pressure and insulin resistance, I recommend that everyone self-monitor themselves for the early signs of these potentially deadly problems. It's easy, and you can do it right in the comfort of your home. And no, you can't leave all of this up to your doctor. Those of you who think that you can wait for your annual check-up are making a terrible mistake. A lot can go wrong in the year or two between visits to the doctor. Procrastination will kill you. Also remember, you are never too young or too old for good health (my residency chairman used to say that).

Why Too Much Insulin Is Very Bad

Big Risk Factor #1: Insulin, *excess* insulin to be specific. Insulin isn't just a risk factor for diabetes. Unhealthy levels of this hormone are a player in both heart attack and stroke, along with a whole host of other diseases. It is crucial for you to acquire an understanding of insulin, the stimuli for its secretion and its bodily effects, some good, others bad.

Insulin is secreted by the pancreas in response to the sugars we eat. It increases the concentration of glucose (sugar) receptors on cell membranes. The receptors subsequently bind the glucose molecules (in the blood) and transport them into the cell. The cell's machinery utilizes glucose to produce ATP (adenosine triphosphate) or cellular energy. In the absence of insulin, one cannot utilize glucose as a fuel source. Remember, for the most part, we are burning either sugar or fat for energy! Juvenile (type I) diabetics secrete little if any insulin, and therefore have to inject the hormone in order to drive sugar into their cells to control blood sugar. Failure to do so WILL result in accelerated aging, early disease onset and potentially death from what is termed ketoacidosis.

Type II diabetes (aka adult onset diabetes) is characterized by **insulin resistance** which is a surplus of circulating insulin. So why are they "diabetic"? It seems counterintuitive. Shouldn't that excess insulin drive sugar into their cells and cause hypoglycemia or low blood sugar? It should yes, *if* one has normal insulin sensitivity. But type II diabetics don't. Their cells are resistant to insulin, resulting in more insulin being required to drive circulating glucose into cells (where it is ultimately oxidized or burned). There is resultant elevation in *both* circulating insulin and blood sugar, *both* of which are pro-inflammatory. More inflammation equates to accelerated aging and early disease onset, right? You see, insulin is toxic to the blood vessel lining, and excess sugar induces the formation of what are referred to as advanced glycation end-products, or AGE's, glucose-protein complexes that accumulate within blood vessel walls. Cumulatively, these two factors narrow blood vessel diameter, ultimately resulting in atherosclerosis. This accelerated atherosclerotic process is the root cause of premature stroke, heart attack and organ (kidney, eye) damage observed in diabetics.

The associated inflammatory state further exacerbates the vascular damage associated with the disease. Diabetes is a *vascular* disease, period. Patients succumb to the vascular complications of the disease (stroke and heart attack for example), NOT to the elevated blood sugar as a discrete entity (except in cases of ketoacidosis). Again, diabetes is a disease that affects the blood vessels. And while it occurs mostly in overweight adults, diabetes can and does occur in individuals with normal body fat levels. So *do not* assume that your fasting blood sugar and your insulin sensitivity are normal just because you're thin. CHECK THEM! How? With a glucometer. These small micro-processor based devices can be purchased inexpensively at virtually every pharmacy. I cannot overstate their value. With one, you can easily gain a handle on your insulin sensitivity and make efforts to optimize it.

You Can Do These Tests At Home

Below, I describe two tests that you can do by yourself at home: a Fasting Blood Sugar (glucose) and a Glucose Tolerance Test. No, you don't need your own at-home laboratory. All you need is a glucometer, a small, portable device about the size of a smartphone that measures the concentration of glucose in the blood. Most of the available glucometers are accurate and highly reliable. All include detailed instructions. Truth be told, they are very simple to use.

1. Fasting blood sugar (glucose):

Your morning finger-stick glucose (after an 8 hour fast). This test is a rough indicator of insulin sensitivity. **Optimal values are 70-85 mg/dL.** We've all been told that "less than 100 is good." That's incorrect. 99 mg/dL is one click away from pre-diabetes.

Even people with modest elevations in fasting glucose (above 85 mg/dL) are at increased risk of a heart attack. This was demonstrated in a study of nearly 2,000 men where fasting blood glucose levels were measured over a 22-year period. Men with fasting glucose over 85 mg/dL had a 40 percent increased risk of death from cardiovascular disease.

You are considered pre-diabetic (insulin resistant) if your fasting serum glucose is > 99 and diabetic if it is > 125 on two serial fasting glucose tests. Either of these conditions places you at elevated risk for vascular disease, and accordingly heart attack, stroke and cancer. And it sneaks up on you! Typically, pre-diabetes (insulin resistance) is asymptomatic. This is precisely why EVERYONE should own a glucometer! It's too late when you've been transported to a local ER having lapsed into a hyperglycemic coma! A glucometer allows for early identification of this potentially lethal disease. Don't hesitate! Buy one today and perform this second test to gain an even better assessment of your insulin sensitivity.

A glucometer allows for early identification of the potentially LETHAL DISEASE, diabetes mellitus.

2. Glucose tolerance test (GTT):

There are numerous studies which demonstrate the harmful effects of elevated postprandial (after-meal) glucose. In fact, poor glucose tolerance (a measure of insulin sensitivity), may result in severe cardiovascular system morbidity seen in diabetics. Part and parcel, there is a direct association between 2 hour postprandial glucose and carotid artery intimal medial thickness (wall thickness), a feature of atherosclerosis. Let me put it in more basic terms: if your 2 hour post-meal blood sugar is elevated, the more likely you are to be damaging your arteries. Similarly, "food comas" are indicative of elevated postprandial blood sugar and elevated insulin levels, both of which are toxins to the endothelium (blood vessel lining).

How efficiently your body clears glucose from your bloodstream (returning blood sugar levels to that of a fasted state) is a direct function of your insulin sensitivity. Insulin is secreted by the pancreas in response to a sugar load (75g in the case of the oral glucose tolerance test for adults). Glucose receptors (cell membrane proteins, with an affinity for the glucose molecule) migrate to the cell surface (from inside the cell) and attach to passerby glucose molecules in the bloodstream. The glucose molecules are then internalized and utilized to generate cellular energy (ATP).

There is dysregulation of this process in the diabetic state. Specifically, glucose transport into the cell is impaired. Such insulin "resistance" causes a reactive hyperinsulinemia (i.e., more insulin is secreted by the pancreas in order to drive glucose into the cell). Again, insulin is toxic to the lining of the blood vessels **and** it stimulates adipogenesis (synthesis and storage of fat), so it is crucial that we maintain *low* levels of circulating insulin chronically. How? By maintaining a high degree of insulin sensitivity. Therefore, for a given sugar load, one would ideally secrete the least possible quantities of insulin to return serum glucose to normal fasting levels.

And how does one maximize insulin sensitivity? Resistance training, stress reduction and proper nutrition, of course. Minimize post-prandial glucose spikes with low glycemic index complex carbohydrates. This will reduce the incidence of "hyperinsulinemic" states, as will adding muscle to your body. And why is muscularity so important? Because muscle, in addition to its role in locomotion and postural maintenance, serves as a depot for both protein and glycogen (a polymerized form of glucose). Glucose is taken up by muscle cells (via the aforementioned receptor-mediated process) in response to its utilization during exercise, specifically intense resistance training. By virtue of this, *muscle serves to lower serum glucose and improve one's insulin sensitivity.* If you hadn't figured it out by now, muscle serves many beneficial *metabolic* roles.

The oral glucose tolerance test does not need to be performed in a doctor's office as you may have been told. And yes, for wondering mothers out there, it is exactly the same test you had while you were pregnant, at the doctor's office. You can easily perform the test at home however, and obtain a baseline to which future studies will be compared. Here's how:

1. After an 8-12 hour fast (during which all medications and supplements are withheld), obtain a baseline glucose level using your glucometer. This is your fasting glucose.

2. Obtain a 75 gram (2/3 cup) glucose drink (readily available online or in select health food stores). Drink the entire solution within a 5 minute period (or less) else the test results will be inaccurate. You are now at "time 0."

3. Test and *record* your blood glucose at time "1 hour."

4. Test and *record* your blood glucose at time "2 hours."

5. Test and *record* your blood glucose at time "3 hours."

NOTE: DO NOT EXERCISE DURING THIS 3-HOUR PERIOD AS THIS WILL AFFECT THE TEST RESULTS.

TEST INTERPRETATION

Parameter	Ideal
Fasting serum glucose	< 86 mg/dL
Glucose, 1 hr. post 75g load	< 140 mg/dL
Glucose, 2 hr. post 75g load	< 120 mg/dL
Glucose, 3 hr. post 75g load	Return to baseline

Remember, the above results are "ideal" or optimal. **Do not panic** if your numbers do not fall into the "ideal" category, but **do something about it!** Why? Because you can! *Type II diabetes is a preventable disease.* Let me mention again, you are considered pre-diabetic (insulin resistant) if your fasting serum glucose is > 99, and diabetic if it is > 125.

It is likely that your glucose tolerance test will be abnormal if your fasting glucose is elevated, as the former is a sign of insulin resistance (barring other confounding factors such as stress and overtraining). Should this be the case, you must seek medical attention. And you must make every effort to improve your insulin sensitivity through proper nutrition (and the associated weight loss), resistance training and stress reduction techniques to name a few.

Remember, diabetes is the underpinning of a variety of lethal diseases, such as coronary artery disease and cancer. Yes, cancer! In this context, does it surprise you that the diabetes drug metformin significantly reduces breast cancer incidence in post-menopausal women? The oral glucose tolerance test may be repeated to monitor your progress. Graph your results (glucose versus time). Shoot for the "ideal" numbers at all hourly points in time.

Understanding the Sugar/Insulin Interaction

As a reader, you may be thinking...

"But I secrete insulin, and my sugar ultimately returns to normal values albeit in a delayed manner. So what's the problem? Why is postprandial glucose important?"

Elevations in post-prandial glucose can have disastrous effects on the vascular wall (endothelium). Regular, chronic elevations in post-prandial glucose cause oxidative stress, the release of inflammatory cytokines (signaling molecules) and promote the formation of advanced glycation end-products (AGEs) with resultant atherosclerosis and arterial narrowing. Acutely, hyperglycemia may induce oxidation of nitric oxide, a potent vasodilator. Restated, *the elevations in blood sugar that occur after a carbohydrate-laden meal may cause destruction of a substance that relaxes our blood vessels.* And this is compounded by the untoward effects of high levels of circulating insulin on vascular relaxation. Have you ever heard of someone having a heart attack or stroke after a heavy meal? Am I making myself clear? Remember this when you're putting that Krispy Kreme donut in your mouth.

Again, how does one go about improving their insulin sensitivity? There seems to be a theme here. Exercise, stress reduction, and proper nutrition! Type II diabetes did not exist 50,000 years ago, I can assure you. It is a *man-made* disease due to unchecked consumption of refined sugar. **Rates of diabetes in 1985 were estimated at 3 million and as of 2010 had reached 28.5 million.** This increase is believed to be due to increasing rates of obesity, stemming from poor nutrition and compounded by outright laziness.

And simple lifestyle modifications work wonders. Consider the Finnish Diabetes Prevention Study, the results of which were published in the New England Journal of Medicine. 522 middle-aged, overweight subjects with impaired glucose tolerance were randomized to intervention and control groups. Each subject in the intervention group received dietary and exercise counseling. Subjects were followed for a mean of 3.2 years.

The incidence of diabetes after four years was 11 percent in the intervention group and 23 percent in the control group. This 58 percent percent reduction in diabetes incidence was directly associated with changes in lifestyle. So it's not as hard as you may think!

Why Track Your Blood Pressure?

Big Risk Factor # 2: High blood pressure, the "silent killer," affects 1/3 of the adult US population. As noted earlier, it is a major risk factor for heart attack and stroke. That's why everyone should own a blood pressure cuff and take their BP at home. It's a cheap piece of home medical equipment that can save your life. Without it, you won't be able to catch high blood pressure in its earliest phase, when simple life style interventions can do the trick.

You don't go from normal BP to high BP overnight. It simply doesn't just 'pop up on you.' The vast majority of cases take years to develop; it slowly creeps up on you. And this to some degree confers protection. How? Because it can be identified early, and it increases in a predictable pattern. Year after year, blood pressure slowly trends upward as arteries stiffen. We know this. This can be tracked and you can intervene early! Prior to your first heart attack.

Hypertension, or high blood pressure, occurs when the resistance to blood flow away from the heart increases. This occurs for a variety of reasons, some of which are genetic, but most are environmental and therefore modifiable. Remember too, that there are very complex interactions between one's genome and the environment; therefore risk factors are not mutually exclusive. Eating a high salt diet does not necessarily mean that you will develop hypertension, contrary to what you have been told—only about 1/3 of the population is salt sensitive. How many people do you know that eat poorly, are obese, yet have normal blood pressure? I know plenty of them. This is clearly due to factors other than the environment (i.e. dietary salt intake).

That being said, we as individuals still have a significant amount of say in where our blood pressure falls on any given day. Those that are "salt sensitive" for example, will respond dramatically to low salt, high potassium diets. Some will not however, requiring a different treatment approach. No matter, the bottom line is that *blood pressure needs to be in check.* As was discussed in the Supplement chapter, the Framingham Study data demonstrated an increasing relation between systolic blood pressure and all-cause, cardiovascular mortality. More simply stated, the higher your blood pressure, the more chances you have of succumbing to a heart attack, period. Seems logical, right? Well it is!

What Is Normal?

Normally, blood pressure should be less than 120/80. Refreshing your memory, the top number, or "systolic", is the pressure in the arteries when the heart beats (when the heart muscle contracts), while the bottom number, or "diastolic", is the pressure in the arteries between heartbeats (when the heart muscle is relaxing between beats and refilling with blood). **Hypertension is defined as serial blood pressure readings of 140/90 or more,** according to the American Heart Association. According to its website, blood pressure screenings should begin at *age 20.* Why? As discussed previously, high blood pressure does not develop overnight. Typically it is years in the making. That being said, **pre-hypertension is defined as systolic pressure of 120-139 or a diastolic of 80-89.** "Or,"rather, one *or* the other. If you qualify as pre-hypertensive based upon serial blood pressure readings, do not take this lightly. This is potentially a harbinger of things to come if left untreated. Deny denial! Blood pressure is an easily tracked and modifiable risk factor once a baseline is established. So, head down to your local pharmacy and purchase a properly fit home blood pressure monitor. I don't care how old you are. Do it!

This next step is very important. I want you to bring the cuff to your doctor's office or to your health care practitioner. Have a member of the medical staff take your blood pressure, as per norm, using the manual cuff. Several minutes later, retake your blood pressure (in the same arm) with the purchased home monitor. Note the differences between both systolic and diastolic *pressures*, between the manual cuff and the home monitor. This is the *offset* or a rough measure of the inaccuracy of your monitor. A manual blood pressure as performed by a trained medical professional, is the most accurate non-invasive measurement, and therefore is considered the gold standard against which your home monitor may be calibrated or standardized.

In light of the inherent inaccuracies of the portable home units, I use them to track trends for the most part. Yes, I am always aware of the offset value and accordingly the blood pressure as an absolute number, but more concerning to me is where my blood pressure is *relative to* where it was. My personal goal is a 110/75. Yours should be similar regardless of age *if* you are currently normotensive. Some of you, women in particular, may have even lower pressures. Good for you! Stay right where you are! Use your monitor on a *weekly* basis and track your blood pressure over time. Chart it. This is not overkill. This is diligence and a requirement for health. Don't assume that a one-time normal blood pressure reading exonerates you from routine surveillance. Remember, arteries stiffen or lose their compliance over time. So get a jump on it, and should your blood pressure start trending upward, consult with your doctor to talk strategy.

HYPERTENSION, PARTICULARLY CHRONIC HYPERTENSION, IS A MAJOR RISK FACTOR FOR STROKE, HEART ATTACK, CONGESTIVE HEART FAILURE, AND PERIPHERAL ARTERIAL DISEASE AND IS A CAUSE OF CHRONIC KIDNEY DISEASE.

Why? Elevations in arterial pressure traumatize the blood vessel lining and promote the development of atherosclerosis. The inciting event in the atherogenic (plaque forming) process is blood vessel injury. By walking around with high blood pressure, you are damaging your arteries! This is akin to the damage inflicted by a high glycemic load meal. In fact, hypertension and diabetes go hand in hand as both diseases afflict severe damage on the vascular system.

Those pre-hypertensive and hypertensive among you (33 percent of American adults have hypertension) have got some work to do. Track your blood pressure *daily*. Aim to normalize your pressure over time; you should know how by now. Those of you on anti-hypertensive medications, attempt to wean yourself off one med at a time (except for maybe an ACE inhibitor or β-blocker). If you are heavy, lose weight. I guarantee you will shed *at least* one medication as your bodyweight normalizes. Case in point is the patient who undergoes bariatric surgery and loses a significant amount of weight. Blood pressure often normalizes obviating the need for medication. This was best exemplified in a study cohort of 1,025 patients who underwent gastric bypass surgery: 66 percent had normalized their blood pressure (and maintained it) at year 5 postoperatively. Interestingly, 86 percent of patients also experienced resolution of diabetes. Resolution! This data suggests that *insulin resistance and hypertension may be indirectly related to each other through the effects of obesity*. In fact, this cluster of risk factors is termed the **Metabolic Syndrome**, or **Syndrome X**. While there are various defining criteria for Metabolic Syndrome, *all* definitions include insulin resistance (impaired glucose tolerance), hypertension and obesity. And these are things that you can test for at home!

High Blood Pressure Can End Badly

Hypertension, particularly chronic hypertension, is a major risk factor for stroke, heart attack, congestive heart failure, peripheral arterial disease and is also a cause of chronic kidney disease. Why? As stated previously, elevations in arterial pressure traumatize the blood vessel lining and promote the development of atherosclerosis. Remember, the inciting event in the atherogenic (plaque forming) process is blood vessel injury. By walking around with high blood pressure, you are damaging your arteries! Let me repeat that, you are damaging your arteries as you read this if your blood pressure is high. This is akin to the damage inflicted by a high glycemic load meal. In fact, hypertension and diabetes go hand and hand as both diseases afflict severe damage on the vascular system.

The vascular damage inflicted by hypertension is *not* what ultimately causes the problem, however. It's the body's *response* to the injury that kills us: atherogenesis or plaque formation. This is a very intricate, multifactorial, inflammatory process. This shouldn't surprise you. Damage invokes inflammation, right? It's a normal response to injury. Consider for a second how the body heals a surgical incision. White blood cells are brought into the area *in response to* chemical messengers released from the injury site (incision). The area is cleaned of debris and growth factors stimulate cellular proliferation. Collagen, the material from which scars are made, is laid down. All this in response to an injury, acutely. So why should the inner lining of a blood vessel be any different? Well, there are some differences (for example, cholesterol is used as the reparative substance) but the processes are very similar. Unfortunately, the end result is narrowing of sometimes crucial blood vessels that supply arterial blood to the heart or brain (the brain, of course is more important to a neurosurgeon). If this narrowing exceeds a critical threshold... heart attack or stroke results respectively.

What is the underpinning of this process? I snuck it in, in the above paragraph, in case you didn't see it. Well, the atherogenic process is no different than any other **pathophysiologic process**. Think hard. *Inflammation*, chronic inflammation. We've discussed how inflammation is a promoter in diseases such as cancer, diabetes and autoimmune processes (lupus and multiple sclerosis, for example). Vascular disease is no different. Arthritis, same thing. And the two are very much related. Think about it. With arthritic processes such as cervical spondylosis (arthritis of the cervical spine or neck), the spinal canal, or tunnels through which the nerves exit the spine, become narrowed. Once this narrowing or stenosis reaches a critical threshold, patients develop symptoms such as pain, weakness or numbness in an extremity, sometimes necessitating surgery. Decompressive spinal surgery is a large part of my practice. Vascular disease, in a similar vein (no pun intended) is manifested as angina or myocardial infarction (heart attack) when it affects the coronary arteries or claudication (leg pain or numbness) when it involves the peripheral blood vessels. You've heard of PAD, right? On those commercials? This stands for P̲eripheral A̲rterial D̲isease. Basically your limbs are becoming ischemic or deprived of needed blood. Muscular demand for oxygen is not being met because of critically narrowed and stiffened blood vessels.

Why? *Chronic* inflammation from chronic vessel wall injury. Treating inflammation with supplements such as omega-3 fatty acids and pharmaceuticals such as aspirin, is integral to the management of both arthritis and vascular disease. And I use them aggressively in my practice. Surgery is a fix when all else fails, but one that is not treating the *etiology* of the disease. Unfortunately, some patients present to the office far along into the disease course and require surgery due to weakness or debilitating pain, for example. This parallels a patient presenting to the ER with crushing chest pain and a first time heart attack. *That* individual is destined for a heart catheterization and most likely an angioplasty. The cat is *long* out of the bag at this point. And why is this? Why are so many afflicted? Heart disease is preventable for the most part. Yes, according to a study performed by the Harvard School of Public Health, "**82 percent** of heart attacks were attributable to failure to follow a healthy lifestyle that includes exercise, good eating habits, and abstinence from smoking." The study cohort of 84,129 women was followed over a period of 14 years.

Whether they knew it or not, the nurses were modifying *modifiable* risk factors, hypertension (and the resultant inflammation) being one of them, through diet and lifestyle choices such as exercise. And you can too! In fact, you have technology at your fingertips which will allow for identification of a multitude of risk factors, many of which can be modified. These include glucometers, smart phone-based exercise and sleep trackers, as well as home blood pressure monitors. This is in addition to the myriad of laboratory tests (discussed in the next chapter) that will allow one to assess for biochemical markers of disease.

The Double Whammy: High BP, High Insulin

The combination of high blood pressure and insulin resistance can lead to Metabolic Syndrome, a condition which affects 44 percent of the U.S. population older than 50. It is bad news at any age. Metabolic Syndrome is associated with a variety of diseases such as type II diabetes, coronary artery disease, PAD, and rheumatic diseases, psoriatic arthritis for example, and aging in general. Does this surprise you? Metabolic Syndrome is simply a cluster of risk factors that, in a synergistic manner, amplify your chances of developing a fatal disease. Its etiology has yet to be elucidated, but as you may have surmised, *inflammation* is suspected to be a major player. This is mediated by the effects of various cellular messengers or cytokines secreted by... fat cells, particularly those that surround your organs. Yet another shocker! Reduce fat, reduce bodily inflammation and reduce your propensity for disease. Are the aspirin and metformin making more sense now?

Whether it's a single disease risk factor or Metabolic Syndrome, do everything in your power to eliminate it. Start with lifestyle modifications such as diet and exercise. Get serious about your health! Do not wait until more risk factors accumulate. Use the home monitors as the barometers of your effort, as your personal guides to treatment. You will notice gradual changes in your fasting (AM) glucose for instance. Check this on a weekly basis. And chart it. Your fasting glucose (and the glucose tolerance test) is a measure of your insulin sensitivity, and to a great degree, *your health*. For most of you, as fat is shed, insulin sensitivity will improve, and so will your waist line. You will *see* the progress right on your glucometer!

Ultimately, technology will allow us to measure far more than blood sugar from the comfort of our home. Detailed biochemical testing will migrate from the doctor's office to your doorstep. The following chapter previews some of the tests that I consider extremely important, tests that will further allow *you* to assume control of *your* health.

METABOLIC Syndrome

We've talked about inflammation and more specifically its role in the genesis of nearly every disease, including diabetes, atherosclerosis, Alzheimer's disease and even cancer. *All diseases share this common link.* Some even fall along a spectrum; literally one disease predisposes you to another. It's a slippery slope with unchecked inflammation as the driving force. There is no better illustration of this than the association of various diseases with the so-called "Metabolic Syndrome" or "Syndrome X."

In actuality, the last sentence should read, "predisposition to" and not "association with." Why? Because if left untreated Metabolic Syndrome is nothing short of a death sentence. While there are various defining criteria for Metabolic Syndrome, *all* definitions include insulin resistance (impaired glucose tolerance), hypertension and obesity. It is a *cluster* of disease processes that act synergistically to decimate not only your body's biochemistry, but also your vascular system. And by now you know what that means...

Metabolic Syndrome—which affects 44 percent of the US population older than 50— is associated with a variety of diseases such as type II diabetes, coronary artery disease, PAD (peripheral artery disease), rheumatic diseases such as psoriatic arthritis and aging in general. As you may have surmised, **inflammation** is suspected to be a major player. Surprising? It shouldn't be. The undercurrent of inflammation is mediated by the effects of various cellular messengers or cytokines secreted by... *fat cells*, particularly those that surround your organs (visceral fat). Another shocker! Reduce fat, reduce bodily inflammation, and reduce your propensity for disease. This equates to longevity! There is a way to measure and actually quantify the amount of inflammation in your body, which I describe in Chapter 10. This basic laboratory test, available to anyone, summarily assesses your body's inner workings and provides critical information. Most importantly, *this information can be acted upon.*

How? By not falling victim to the perils of obesity and in particular insulin resistance (IR). Shedding fat with exercise and good nutrition will dampen the flames of inflammation scalding your body's innards. I wouldn't be telling you this in such graphic language if it was hopeless! Far from it. Even small steps taken in the right direction can make a big difference. If you are obese, strive for a 10 percent weight loss over a period of six months. By doing so, you will dramatically improve your insulin sensitivity as evidenced in a 2004 study of bariatric surgical patients. Not only were the features of the Metabolic Syndrome improved among the study cohort, but *95.6 percent of patients were cured.* The implications of this study are monumental. Think about it. How many diseases are linked o, associated with, or potentiated by Metabolic Syndrome? A boatload. Logic would suggest therefore that *a very effective way to prevent age-related disease is to maintain body fat levels within the normal range*. In fact, I would strive for the low end of the normal range as provided by the National Strength and Conditioning Association (NSCA). Shedding fat will also improve your insulin sensitivity and likely reduce your blood pressure significantly. The impact on your health cannot be overstated.

Unfortunately, despite global awareness of Metabolic Syndrome and its potentially devastating consequences, its prevalence is on the rise. According to the National Health and Nutrition Examination Survey, the incidence of obesity in the United States has increased from 13.4 percent to 34.3 percent from 1960-2008. And this is despite significant advancements in medical technology coupled with a better understanding of human pathophysiology. So why are we so fat and *growing* fatter? You don't need to be a brain surgeon to answer this question! The answer is as simple as it is obvious. We are getting sicker because of inactivity, poor dietary choices and limited health education. Physical education in schools, if anything, has been de-emphasized in recent years. What type of message is this sending to our children? I know... that daily exercise is *not* a vital element in the maintenance of health and well-being. That we don't

need to be physically active. Concomitant with the decline in PE requirements has been the rise in childhood obesity. The prevalence of obesity *quadrupled* over 25 years among boys and girls, making them ripe for the development of Metabolic Syndrome and its associated consequences. And the gaming industry has flourished as our children become less able to fit into an airplane seat.

Get your children off their asses! The effects of physical activity are far-reaching. Once an individual incorporates exercise into his daily regimen, it becomes an integral part of his or her life. There simply is no better preventive strategy especially if such "physicality" is coupled with sound diet and nutrition. And the data suggests just that. "Higher moderate-to vigorous-intensity physical activity (MVPA) time by children and adolescents was associated with better cardiometabolic risk factors regardless of the amount of sedentary time," according to a recent study that appeared in the prestigious *Journal of the American Medical Association* (JAMA). In English? *Exercise is protective of the body.*

Metabolic Syndrome is your arch nemesis, literally priming the body for the many age-related diseases discussed in this text. So follow my lead and prevent yourself from becoming that "ticking time-bomb" awaiting your first bout of crushing chest pain.

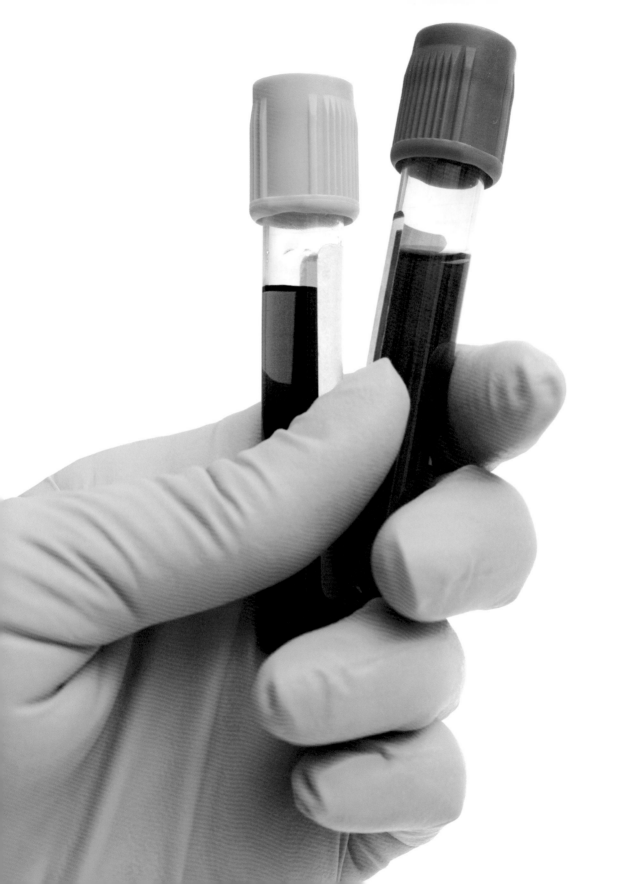

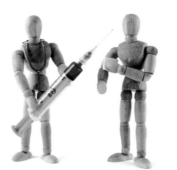

BLOOD TESTS

Knowing your risk factors for disease is an essential first step towards prevention. It is nearly impossible to achieve optimal health without taking intermittent snapshots of the inner workings of your body to guide you, which can be provided by laboratory testing.

TO INSIST ON

Relatively inexpensively, *your* biochemistry can be accurately assessed and potential disease risk factors identified. As you make strides to improve your insulin sensitivity or blood pressure, you can also lower serum inflammatory markers and optimize your lipid profile. But first you must establish a baseline to which future testing may be compared. Below are five tests that I consider important *in the context of age-related disease*, or more simply put, those diseases that will kill you dead.

LIPID PROFILE

This test is used to determine total cholesterol and quantifies HDL, LDL and triglycerides. Basic lipid profile testing provides a rough idea of the ratio of "good" to "bad" cholesterol. With regard to LDL in particular, more important than the absolute number, is "particle size" or "subtype." This may be determined by a VAP test. More on this later.

HDL or high-density lipoprotein is a scavenger of LDL (low-density lipoprotein) which is found in atherosclerotic plaques. HDL binds and transports LDL back to the liver for recycling. Please keep in mind that it is the *oxidized* LDL that is atherogenic, which means it has the potential to cause damage to the inner lining of our arteries. A primary cause of coronary artery disease, LDL unto itself is harmless. The body's natural antioxidant systems can be easily overloaded, however, with resultant accumulation of oxidized LDL in the vascular endothelium (and hence plaque formation). This is one reason why it is critical to support the body's antioxidant system with supplements. Better still, attempt to maintain LDL near 100 mg/dL and HDL over 50 mg/dL in order to minimize any potential for oxidized particles to become incorporated into the blood vessel lining.

Having obtained your test results, do not become preoccupied with your cholesterol/triglyceride values *if* your other vascular risk factors are minimized. Why? First, be aware of the fact that a significant percentage of patients undergoing coronary bypass surgery have _____ (you fill in the blank) cholesterol.

Answer: NORMAL!

So there are other critical risk factors for coronary artery disease. The 2004 INTERHEART study identified those risk factors, and guess what? All are modifiable: ApoB/apoA1 (an indirect measure of LDL/HDL ratio), smoking, diabetes, hypertension, abdominal obesity, psychosocial, daily consumption of fruits and vegetables, exercise and alcohol intake. So where is TOTAL cholesterol (so often considered a crucial marker for coronary disease)? Let's see... NOWHERE.

Remember too that cholesterol is the "mother of all hormones," the precursor to hormones such as cortisol, progesterone, testosterone and estradiol. We *need* cholesterol. So don't strive to "fix the number" just because it may be abnormally elevated. Instead, improve your cholesterol profile by optimizing the above ratios through sound nutrition, exercise and potentially supplements (e.g. omega-3 fatty acids and niacin).

As you take these simple steps to improve your cholesterol, you will note a decrease in your triglyceride level. What are triglycerides? Simple. Blood borne fats that are affixed to a carrier molecule of glycerol, hence the name. Patients routinely tell me that their diets are "excellent" or that "they don't eat a lot." I get an entirely different story from their triglyceride levels, which are a direct reflection of their diets. Excessive consumption of refined carbohydrates and animal fats equates to high triglycerides, period. The proof is in the blood. Your serum triglyceride level serves as a looking glass into your gut. I know what you've been eating...

Logic dictates therefore that an optimal (under 100 mg/dL) triglyceride level is associated with eating less sugar and inflammatory fat. Independent of triglyceride level, these two dietary modifications confer protection against age-related disease. You know that. Conversely, an elevation in serum triglyceride, in particular when associated with lowered HDL, is a potential harbinger of disaster. An unfavorable ratio of triglyceride to HDL essentially primes the body for plaque formation. In fact, this ratio is a proven independent risk factor for coronary disease. If your triglyceride: HDL ratio is > 4, you're in trouble. Shoot for an ideal ratio of 2.

VAP TESTING

Now, a couple of words on **VAP testing**. The **V**ertical **A**uto **P**rofile is a cholesterol, lipid and lipoprotein test. It measures all the components of a standard lipid profile but delves further, segmenting cholesterol into subclasses. Subtype A is "fluffy" and less apt to be integrated into atherosclerotic plaque, while subtype B is dense and atherogenic. A standard lipid profile *does not* differentiate the two. For this reason, it is completely erroneous to assume that elevations in LDL are wholly bad. Your LDL may be composed mainly of subtype A. Interestingly, lower triglyceride levels are associated with higher levels of this subtype, while higher triglyceride levels are associated with the smaller, denser type B particles.

Secondarily, VAP testing quantifies your lipoprotein(a), or Lp(a) cholesterol level. Elevated serum levels of this LDL-like particle are an independent risk factor for coronary artery and cerebrovascular disease. Similar to oxidized LDL, lipoprotein(a) accumulates in the endothelium during the atherogenic process. Understandably, elevated levels are seen in patients with carotid artery plaque and resultant arterial narrowing, an obvious risk factor for stroke. Interestingly, the physiologic role of Lp(a) has yet to be fully discovered. We do know that low levels typically equate to vascular health, while elevated levels are associated with ER visits.

I would strongly consider VAP testing *in lieu* of the standard lipid profile if you have high blood pressure, diabetes or a family history of heart disease or stroke. *Basically if you are at risk, default to VAP testing.* You may be surprised to learn that what was once deemed "normal" in the standard lipid profile (i.e. LDL), is far from it.

CRP (HIGH-SENSITIVITY)

Remember when we talked about the relationship between gum disease and coronary heart disease incidence? What was the link between the two? Chronic *Inflammation.* You knew that was coming. In fact, several small cohort studies demonstrated the efficacy of antibiotics in reducing atherosclerosis. What? Yes, reducing the chronic inflammation associated with gingival disease thwarts the atherogenic process. By no means am I recommending haphazard usage of antibiotics, rather, I am telling you to have your CRP checked. Flossing daily may help too.

CRP or C-reactive protein is what is known as an "acute phase reactant." It is a protein secreted by the liver in response to a variety of stimuli, namely those which activate the inflammatory cascade. Interestingly, one of the factors that cause an elevation in CRP levels is secreted by adipocytes or fat cells. It should not come as a surprise therefore to learn that patients with Metabolic Syndrome, a premorbid condition associated with a variety of diseases, have elevated CRP levels. In fact, CRP is an independent risk factor for coronary heart disease, hypertension, type II diabetes and atherogenic dyslipidemia.

Elevations in hsCRP are no joke. Take them seriously! Do not procrastinate and allow bodily inflammation to run rampant one day longer. Stop inflamm-aging in its tracks with proper nutrition, exercise, supplements, and, if need be, pharmaceuticals. *Drive your hsCRP down to zero.* This is an indication that you are doing something right...

HOMOCYSTEINE

Similar to CRP, elevations in homocysteine are associated with a variety of disease entities such as heart attack, stroke, Alzheimer's disease and osteo-porosis. Homocysteine is an intermediary in a complex series of biochemical reactions that play a role in neurotransmitter (chemicals that allow nerve cells to communicate with one another) synthesis and DNA methylation (regulation of gene expression). It can accumulate in the blood for several reasons, the most common of which is vitamin B deficiency (as several of the aforementioned reactions are dependent on the presence of vitamin B). In fact, almost two-thirds of the prevalence of high homocysteine is attributable to low vitamin status or intake.

There are two issues here to consider. First, the build-up of homosysteine suggests that critical biochemical pathways (noted above) are faltering. It should be present in low levels in the plasma. Methylation is otherwise impaired and a variety of inflammatory diseases (as above) set in. Even fatigue and depression can be due to methylation defects! Secondly, and adding insult to injury, homocysteine itself is an endothelial toxin; it wreaks havoc on your blood vessels. Again, you are only as old as your blood vessels are.

The good thing? Elevated levels of homocysteine are easily addressed even in patients with genetic predispositions to what are termed "methylation defects." I'll spare you the details. Simply, take a B-complex vitamin daily as recommended. In the event that your serum homocysteine level still is not maintained between 5 and 8 micromols/L, add 800 mcg of daily folic acid, 1000 mcg of vitamin B12, 30 mg of zinc, and 100 mg of vitamin B6 daily. Some individuals may require 500 mg of daily trimethylglycine (TMG) as well. These are all readily available at your local health food store. You heard me, *over-the-counter products can save your life.*

HEMOGLOBIN A1C

You may have heard about "A1c" levels. So what's the deal? It's easy to understand really. Hemoglobin, the oxygen carrying iron-based protein within your red blood cells, can become "glycosylated," as can other bodily proteins in the formation of AGE's, or advanced glycosylation end-products. Remember those? They're bad. High levels of HbA1c are similarly bad.

Glucose (sugar) molecules irreversibly bind to a protein subunit of hemoglobin in a predictable manner that is directly proportional to serum glucose levels. In English: *persistent elevations in serum glucose raise HbA1c levels.* Why is this important? Glycosylated hemoglobin levels reflect *long-term* blood sugar levels. It is an indication of how well your blood sugar has been controlled over weeks to months. This test doesn't lie. It is an average, a wide-angle lens, not an instantaneous snapshot like a fasting glucose level. For this reason, it is a more accurate reflection of one's insulin sensitivity. And you know how important that is...

So what should your A1c level be? My answer? As low as possible... As your body (particularly your brain) relies on glucose for energy (ATP) production, it is physiologically impossible to drive your A1c level to zero. Your body has very effective biochemical mechanisms to maintain blood sugar within a certain range. To fuel your brain! By virtue of this, a percentage of your red blood cells' hemoglobin will be glycosylated. Normal blood sugars yield an HbA1c level of 4.5-5 percent. One is considered diabetic (by the American Diabetes Association) if HbA1c is 6.5 percent or greater. Keep these numbers in mind and strive for five or less through proper nutrition, resistance training, and stress reduction techniques. Follow your fasting glucose at home; *persistently* low levels will ultimately translate to normal HbA1c (and hopefully longevity).

VITAMIN D₃

As discussed previously, vitamin D_3 is a vital hormone involved in hundreds of biologic processes. Until relatively recently, its importance was underappreciated. Yes, we were aware of its effects on bone health and calcium regulation, and yes, we knew that it was produced when one's skin was exposed to ultraviolet radiation. But *now*, we are aware of its wide array of benefits (and I mean wide). You see, vitamin D_3 receptors have been identified on many cell types including those of the heart and the brain. *Its presence is required for normal cell function.* Knowing this, why is it that so many Americans are vitamin D_3 deficient? It boils down to two things really: lack of awareness of its health-promoting effects *and* poor surveillance. Whatever the case may be, do not hesitate. Get tested and intervene if necessary, as *failure to do so will predispose you to a variety of diseases.*

Why is the knowledge of your vitamin D_3 level so critical? There is evidence that Vitamin D_3 deficiency is associated with stroke, insulin resistance, Alzheimer's dementia, coronary artery disease and cancer. So supplement aggressively, and strive for a serum level of 50-65 ng/mL. Do not for a second assume that the RDA of 600 International Units (I.U.'s) is sufficient. It's not (unless you literally *live* in the sun). Similarly, do not rely on a daily glass of "fortified" milk to satisfy your daily vitamin D_3 requirements. That's a joke. The

100 plus I.U.'s supplied per eight-ounce glass is a drop in the bucket relative to your needs. I take 10,000 units daily to maintain my level of near 65 ng/mL. Take it from me, *your levels are suboptimal.* Don't believe me? Go get tested, I'll prove it to you...

Note:

Hormone panels (i.e. thyroid function tests) and replacement therapy (HRT) will be discussed in chapter 11. Keep in mind too, that there is a myriad of laboratory tests, many of which are esoteric, available to you. I would *not* recommend a shotgun approach however; do not subject yourself to every laboratory test under the sun. *The above are excellent screening tests, the results of which you will potentially **act** upon. They may change your life. Insist that your doctor orders them.*

EST AND

DENTIFY YOUR RISK FACTORS FOR DISEASE.

ODIFY OR

LIMINATE YOUR RISK FACTORS.

E-TEST.

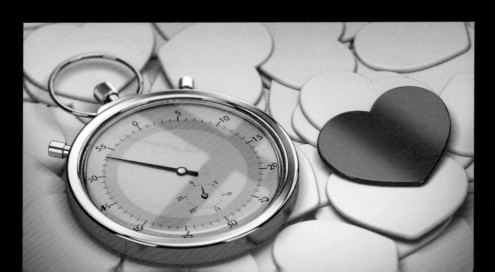

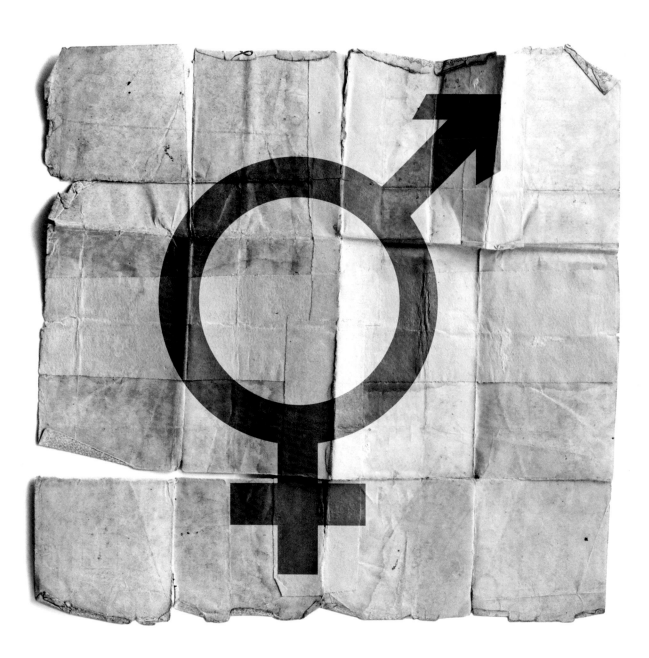

the TRUTH about HORMONES

Remember how great you felt when you were 18? Your mind was clear, your attitude carefree, and you were ready to take on the world. You were motivated and full of enthusiasm (and likely libido). You were bursting with energy. And you were far stronger, leaner, and mentally sharper than you are now. You wish you had that back, right? Who doesn't? What happened to all that vim and vigor?

Life happened. Humans have a finite life expectancy of course, as the mysteries of aging, the *disease* of aging has yet to be elucidated. At this point, we cannot prevent the body from aging, but we can thwart the process to some degree. And while there is undoubtedly a genetic component to aging, it is likely that it too is related to the accumulation of metabolic by-products within our cells, like oil residue within our car's cylinders.

You see, everything you do to some degree, is putting mileage on the odometer. There are toxic metabolic by-products and free radicals generated even during the *digestive* process, for example. That's why aging is inescapable! That being said, *good* nutrition and more specifically foods loaded with antioxidants will quench those free radicals formed during meals, to some degree hindering the aging process. Exercise as well bolsters antioxidant status, as was discussed previously. Those not overtraining typically maintain their youthful appearance, right? To a great degree, this is related to the beneficial effects of exercise on one's hormones. Exercise not only makes you look great but *feel* great!

18 Again?

Exercise has the *potential* to restore hormones, particularly growth hormone and testosterone, to their youthful levels. Truth-be-told however, this occurs in only a minority of individuals for a variety of reasons. Stress wreaks havoc on the endocrine system for example, countering the effects of exercise. No sleep? The damage is compounded further as cortisol (stress hormone) levels rise and sex hormones plummet. Fatigued, flabby, and forty, you no longer can keep up with your children. But there is hope: HRT or hormone replacement therapy.

I know, you've heard that hormones are dangerous, and more specifically that they *cause* cancer. That if you take testosterone for example, you're *destined,* as a male, to develop prostate cancer. Nothing could be further from the truth! This is a myth. No, it's an outright lie. If taking testosterone causes prostate cancer, then why don't all adolescent males develop the disease? Their hormones are raging, right? Damn right. This claim therefore defies logic and well… reality.

Estrogen and progesterone have fallen under similar scrutiny. The merits and flaws of the Women's Health Initiative (WHI) study however will not be discussed here, as they are outside the scope of this book. Suffice it to say that many women are being deprived of **bio-identical** hormone replacement therapy, which not only can improve quality of life, but also prevent osteoporosis and its associated morbidities. Part of the problem stemmed from the fact that *oral* estrogen was utilized in the WHI study, as opposed to a transdermal preparation. *Transdermal* estrogens, on the other hand, are *not* metabolized by the liver and *do not* appear to increase the risk of blood clots according to the recent Kronos Early Estrogen Prevention Study (KEEPS). So stop the madness people! Do not make rash medical decisions based on a flawed study. Instead, discuss the option of HRT with your doctor. It's not for everyone, but can make a dramatic difference in the lives of those that opt in.

How do you know if you're a candidate? Good question. Men are easy, women a bit more complicated, particularly *pre*-menopausal women. Yes, they too are eligible for HRT; it's not just for women with hot flashes. In fact, *progesterone* levels start declining at around age 35, before estrogen! And there are many manifestations of progesterone deficiency: abnormal menses, headaches, depression, mood swings, insomnia and loss of bone mineral density to name a few. Experienced any of these? Most women have. And they're treated with Advil, Prozac, and Ambien; hormone deficiency is rarely considered. It certainly wasn't part of my medical school curriculum.

We *did however* learn that the prostate is a hormone sensitive gland. Testosterone in particular, was vilified in the context of prostate cancer. It "*caused*" prostate cancer. In actuality, elevated levels of *estrogen,* not testosterone, may play a major role in the genesis of prostate cancer. And guess what happens to estrogen levels in males as they age? They increase! Males assume the hormone profile of a female as they get older. **Testosterone plummets as estrogen levels rise**. Does your husband or boyfriend have "man boobs?" This is often times a function of elevated estrogen levels.

In women, estrogen, progesterone and testosterone levels fall, placing them at risk for age-related disease as their risk for developing heart disease and related conditions accumulate. This decline can be tempered by hormone replacement therapy, the goal of which is two-fold: restoration *and* balance. And this is where medicine becomes equally an art, as it is a science. It is sometimes tricky to balance one's hormones and, often times, requires trial and error (and patience). Your hormonal regimen will likely be different from that of your sister. Although you may look alike, her biochemistry is *undoubtedly* distinct from yours. While you may feel great with a certain dosage and frequency of transdermal estrogen, she may be unresponsive to *that particular* regimen, or she may have undesired side effects. It's not about restoring blood hormone levels to "normal." Normal estradiol levels span a wide range. That being said, your optimal level may be on the opposite end of the "normal" spectrum than that of your sister. Who cares? *How you feel* is much more important than the actual hormone level. This requires that all important body-mindfulness I've spoken about. *You must be in touch with your body, and your doctor must be responsive to your needs.*

The same is true for men. Men have it a bit easier though, go figure. Estrogen and progesterone typically are not much of a concern, so there is no balancing act. Males typically respond very well to restoration of serum testosterone levels and concomitant lowering of estradiol. Bring one up, the other down and voilà, a biochemical restoration of a youthful hormone profile, and often times, a new lease on life. As mentioned above, men too have to be on the same page as their doctors. Hormones *do* have side effects, although they can be minimized, if not eliminated, by providing your doctor with accurate feedback. An open communication line is mandatory *prior* to the start of a hormone replacement regimen.

So How Do I Get Started?

Provided you meet clinical criteria, your doctor will order a battery of blood tests which will measure a variety of hormone levels. These are your baseline levels to which future results will be compared. I typically draw hormone panels every 6-12 weeks initially, and upon optimizing the patient, every 3-6 months thereafter. A hormone panel for a female may include the following:

Estradiol

Total Estrogen

Progesterone

Total and Free Testosterone

Sex Hormone Binding Globulin (SHBG)

TSH

Free T3 and T4

DHEA-S

Cortisol

IGF-I

Your physician will design a restorative regimen based on your test results and symptoms. This will likely include dietary modifications, exercise, supplements, and hormone preparations.

Hormones come in all shapes and sizes, but not all are created equal. Some, in fact, are associated with significant risks. In that regard, I give you two cardinal rules:

RULE #1

Use only **BIO-IDENTICAL** hormone preparations. Synthetic hormones (i.e. progest*ins*) are dangerous, plain and simple. The fact that progest*in* was utilized in the WHI study (as opposed to bio-identical progest*erone*) was an overt flaw in the study design, which ultimately deprived many women of the potential benefits of HRT. ***Progestins are not progesterone***. Do you know any women who have developed "blood clots" from birth control pills? Progest*ins* at work.

RULE #2

AVOID oral testosterone and oral estrogens. The breakdown products (metabolites) of both testosterone and estrogen are potentially carcinogenic. I would recommend transdermal (cream) preparations for each. Progesterone may be taken orally or compounded into a cream as well. Testosterone may be injected intramuscularly. The specific route of administration will be determined by your physician.

Don't Be Stupid

Hormone replacement therapy carries with it the stigma of danger, unjustified danger. While HRT is not for everyone (those with a strong family history of hormone sensitive cancers, for example), *many potential candidates are never even given the option.* And this is nothing short of ignorance among members of the medical field. Sheer stupidity.

Speaking of stupidity, allow me to tell you a quick story. An old friend of the family had been referred to me, not for a neurosurgical issue, but for a recent alteration in personality and memory loss. I agreed to see her by virtue of our relationship, but ultimately intended to refer her to a neurology colleague for a formal workup. Based on her description over the phone (prior to her office visit), it appeared as if this 61-year-old potentially was developing an early *dementia.* She complained of short term memory loss and she wasn't as sharp. Her affect had changed as well, and she was unable to "find happiness." More concerning was the fact that she had been told by friends that she was "acting funny" and frankly "stupid."

I found her to be completely normal neurologically. There were no symptoms suggestive of a brain tumor such as headache, nausea, vomiting, or weakness. The mental changes she described had been present for approximately three months and were fairly sudden in onset. There was no history of head trauma or infection. But you want to

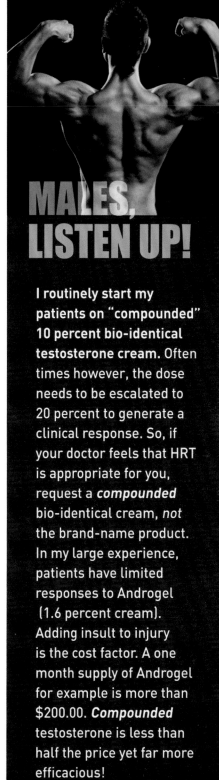

MALES, LISTEN UP!

I routinely start my patients on "compounded" 10 percent bio-identical testosterone cream. Often times however, the dose needs to be escalated to 20 percent to generate a clinical response. So, if your doctor feels that HRT is appropriate for you, request a *compounded* bio-identical cream, *not* the brand-name product. In my large experience, patients have limited responses to Androgel (1.6 percent cream). Adding insult to injury is the cost factor. A one month supply of Androgel for example is more than $200.00. *Compounded* testosterone is less than half the price yet far more efficacious!

know the most interesting thing that I teased out of her upon questioning? *This had happened before.* Twice, in fact. When? When she was 16 *and* just after the birth of her daughter. The exact same feeling, and she had lived her life fearful that *the feeling* would recur. And it did. Hmm...

So what do these three episodes have in common? The former episodes both occurred during periods of wild hormonal fluctuation, right? Ever hear of "post-partum depression?" It's been all over the news. This syndrome is thought to be related to an acute drop in the mother's *progesterone* levels after giving birth. But my patient was post-menopausal; gone were the hormonal swings of youth. If anything, her estrogen levels were relatively static, as she was on transdermal estradiol. But what about *progesterone*? It wasn't on her medication list.

"Were you *ever* on supplemental progesterone?" I asked, noting the similarity between all *three* episodes.

She said, "I tried this non-prescription progesterone cream in the past, but didn't feel anything. I used it for about a year."

"Really," I said. "When did you stop it?"

"About **three** months ago," she replied.

And when did these recent symptoms start again?" I asked.

"About **three** months ago..."

I started my patient on nightly bio-identical progesterone to correct the hormonal imbalance. Her mental state, memory, and depression improved dramatically, nearly returning to baseline within three **weeks.** Point being?.... Do not underestimate the roles that hormones play in your biochemistry, and more specifically, in your well-being. Progesterone exerts very important effects on the nervous system, as was just demonstrated. In fact, it is being used successfully as a neuroprotective agent in head-injured patients, in both women and men. Both women AND men! Yes, men too *need* progesterone. Some researchers have even proposed that Alzheimer's disease is in part due to progesterone deficiency. We all may be on some form of HRT one day.

In this light, I would urge you to explore the option of hormone replacement therapy with your doctor. Restoring a youthful hormone profile not only has the potential to make you feel great, but also may impede the aging process. The question still remains, do our hormone levels decline as we age, or do we age *as a result of* our declining hormone levels? Chicken or the egg? My bet is on the latter...

The Steroid Hormone Cascade

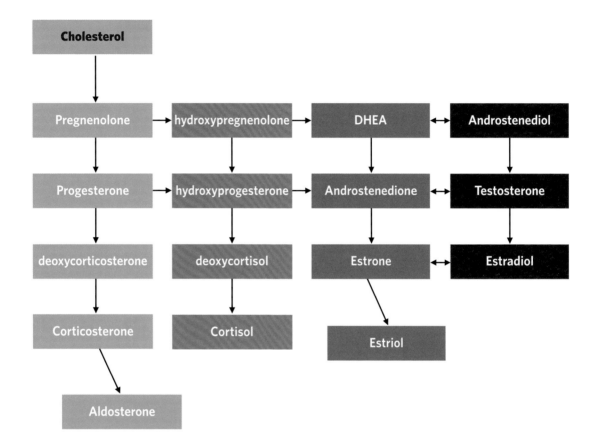

Remember, *cholesterol* is the "mother" of all hormones (statin users beware!). It is the precursor of cortisol and the sex hormones testosterone, estrogen and progesterone, which by virtue of their common origin, are interrelated. But it's more than a "relationship;" it's a balance, a **critical balance.** Hormonal balance is associated with health, while lack thereof is associated with disease. Vigorous exercise, proper nutrition and stress reduction techniques tip the scales in favor of a balanced, youthful hormone profile. Along with that, come a sharper mind, a more shapely body, better sex and increased energy levels. Any takers?

THE
STRENGTH
TRAINING PROTOCOL

I give you what has worked best for
me over the past 30 years…

In Chapter 5 you were introduced to the basic and foundational movements of the strength training protocol that I use. In my opinion (one shared by many others), these exercises will time after time provide you with the greatest gains from the standpoint of muscularity and strength. They are the staples of both powerlifters and bodybuilders. There is no argument in this regard. Of much debate, however, is the optimal way to organize your training regimen. In truth, there are myriads of "systems" out there claiming to be the best. And most work—for most people, some of the time. But what if you are in the minority for whom the regimen fails? What then? And why did that particular program fail to live up to its claims? Well, it's not the *program* per se, it is failed introspection. If I can leave you with one message in this regard, always default to your sense of "body mindfulness." Follow the outlined protocol for at least six months and assess your physical and strength gains frequently. Assure that your nutrition is optimal, and that you are getting adequate rest. **Make training a priority.** And don't quit if you're not making

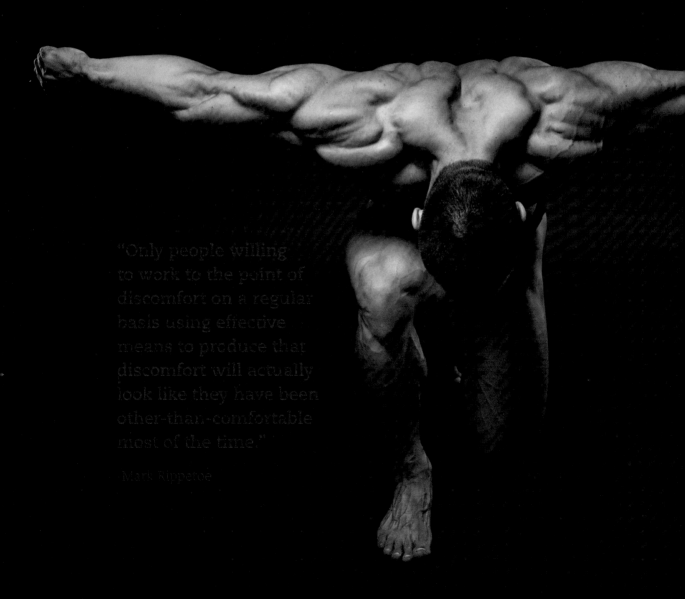

Appendix

(and deltoids, rhomboids, and trapezius)

"Only people willing
to work to the point of
discomfort on a regular
basis using effective
means to produce that
discomfort will actually
look like they have been
other-than-comfortable
most of the time."

–Mark Rippetoe

the progress that you hoped for. Instead, persevere! Reassess the variables that may be impeding your progress. Better your nutrition. Get more sleep. Add an additional rest day as needed. Look deep inside, and do not be afraid to experiment. Your body will respond given time. *Establish what works best for you.*

That being said, I give you what has worked best for **me** over the past 30 years...

The following program targets the predominant muscle fiber types, type I, type IIa, and type IIb. Viewed another way, the program stresses the dominant energy systems of the body. It's a feat of strength to be able to squat 405 lbs.—but can you sprint up 10 flights of stairs without developing chest pain? Therein lies the problem with isolated training. The program that I utilize develops strength and muscular endurance but does not exclude a pure "steady-state" endurance workout on account of its proven cardiovascular benefits. And in addition, the endurance training will provide not only a "fat-burning" effect, but also serve as a respite for your heavily taxed muscles.

This program makes sense.

I challenge you to walk into any gym and observe your surroundings. I find the routine demonstrations of irrational exercise quite amusing. The majority of individuals possess little knowledge of exercise or the mechanics of the exercises they are performing! They are simply going through the motions in the hopes of appeasing Hercules. Is this you? Or do you fall into the category of people who refer to *Muscle and Fitness* for exercise advice? Please listen to me. You are being misled. Bilked! Muscle magazines are nothing more than advertisement forums for supplement companies. A glorified sales pitch. An unreliable source of information on par with the "gym rat" that continues to make drug-induced gains *despite* his/her exercise regimen.

Science, and science only, governs and dictates the principles of strength training. The layperson, often times *regardless* of his/her physique, has little knowledge of said principles. Take a look around. A large percentage of techniques utilized in modern-day facilities are baseless. Only a select few are training properly, with high intensity, and intensity enough to stimulate growth of that sought-after muscle. Statistically you are *not* among them, having failed to make any significant physical gains despite years of "working out." Well, it's time for a change! This change of thought and a functional understanding of exercise science will vault you to new levels of health, strength, and physical appearance. Stop wasting your time! Don't follow the masses. Instead follow your logic.

What follows is a logical training protocol from which YOU will formulate one best suited to YOUR fitness goals. If you are an endurance athlete, you may consider dropping the mid-week "strength-endurance" session. Do not forego the resistance training however. Instead, **make it a priority.** I promise you, it will dramatically improve your performance and give you that competitive edge. I'm talking to you Ms. Cyclist...

The program is elegant in its simplicity. There is really nothing fancy about it. I summarize it this way:

Day	Modality
Monday & Friday	Strength
Tuesday & Thursday	Steady-State Endurance
Wednesday	Strength-Endurance

Huh?

Allow me to explain...

Training is done five days per week. Weekends are *completely* off. This will allow for bodily recovery and muscular growth. Training is a significant stress to the body. Allow it to recover. Else risk stalled progress or worse: overtraining syndrome.

Training sessions will take no more than 1 hour each. You are otherwise moving too slowly and thereby reducing training intensity. *Intensity* is one of the prerequisites for neuromuscular response to a training stimulus. Intensity refers to the energy expenditure during exercise or more simply, how hard you are working. Those sessions dedicated to **Strength** on both Monday and Friday, will be of fairly high intensity based upon weight utilized. The midweek session of **Strength-Endurance** will be of similar intensity by virtue of the short rest utilized between movements, and the moderate weight loads. If you wear a heart rate monitor during your training, you will note fairly similar numbers on Monday, Wednesday, and Friday, as heart rate is a direct correlate of intensity. In fact, there are training programs based wholly on heart rate.

Cyclists and rowers typically utilize such schemes specifically to improve their sprinting abilities, training at the so called "lactate threshold." **Steady-State Endurance** work in this protocol however is of far less intensity and therefore associated with lower heart rates. The relative low intensity of Tuesday and Thursday's endurance sessions allows the body to recover from preceding high intensity sessions.

WEEKLY INTENSITY SCHEMA:

Monday	Tuesday	Wednesday	Thursday	Friday
High	Low	Med-High	Low	High

Makes sense, doesn't it?
Again, weekends are completely off. Intensity level: ZERO. No discussion.

Let's delve a little deeper to better your understanding of the protocol. The varied intensities utilized in the protocol (as above) stress different energy systems and muscle fiber types. No stone is left unturned in your quest for *comprehensive* fitness.

Low intensity training or **Steady-State Endurance,** targets the type I muscle fibers which rely on oxidative phosphorylation of fatty acids ("fat burning") for production of ATP (cellular energy).

High intensity training on **Strength** day targets type IIb muscle fibers to a great degree (all fibers are actually recruited sequentially). These "fast-twitch" fibers rely on the "phosphocreatine" and "glycolytic" systems for ATP production, because these biochemical processes rapidly provide ATP for muscle contraction. How else could grandma lift the car off the pinned child? With oxidative type I or "slow twitch" fibers? I think not. Similarly, heavy deadlifts will stress your type IIb fibers. These are the fibers that give your muscles their shape.

Midweek, **Strength-Endurance** work will target the type IIa muscle fibers predominantly. These fibers are "oxidative-glycolytic," a sort of hybrid of type I and type II fibers. They are "fast-twitch" yet rely on oxidative phosphorylation and glycolysis for ATP production. These fibers fatigue faster than type I fibers although slower than type IIb fibers (which fatigue extremely rapidly).

Keep in mind that these are not absolutes. In other words, workouts are not targeting a *single* fiber type. You can't! Muscles are composed of several fiber types (more than mentioned above) and all are firing to some degree during heavy lifts in particular. This has to do with "recruitment" patterns and is not germane to the discussion. Suffice it to say that low intensity exercise stresses the type I, slow-twitch fibers, and more demanding, exhausting tasks *preferentially* target type II fibers. This will make more sense when the entire protocol is laid out.

SCHEMATICALLY:

Day	Monday	Tuesday	Wednesday	Thursday	Friday
Intensity	High	Low	Med-High	Low	High
Fiber Type	Type IIb	Type I	Type IIa	Type I	Type IIb
Energy System	PCr, Glycolysis	Ox Phos	Ox-Gly	Ox Phos	PCr, Glycolysis

PCr = Phosphocreatine   Ox Phos = Oxidative phosphorylation
Ox-Gly = Oxidative phosphorylation and Glycolysis

That's it! *Alternating* workouts. *Alternating* energy systems and fiber types. **All** *addressed.*

So how do you incorporate the foundational movements into the scheme? How are the sessions structured? Easy. Let's begin with the **Strength** days, Monday and Friday.

PROTOCOL GUIDELINES

1. **Squatting is paired with overhead press.**
   They are performed on the same day albeit at different intensities.

2. **Deadlifting is paired with bench press.**

---

3. **5 x 5 protocol** is utilized except when performing deadlifts (3 x 5). This is a well-described, time-tested resistance training protocol geared toward the development of **Strength** (using approximately 85 percent of your

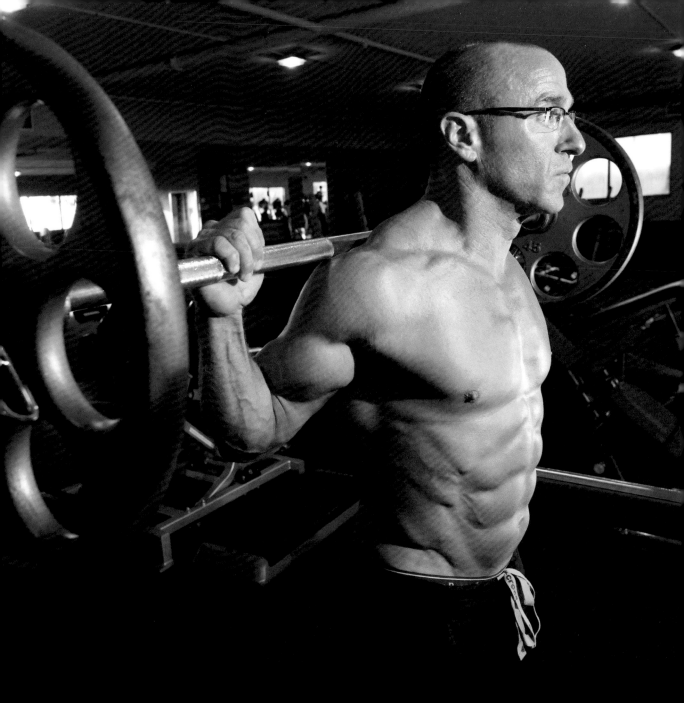

People often ask me how to get **big biceps**.
My answer: "Squats!" A strong mid-section? Same answer.
Just see for yourself. There is no posing here. By *virtue of
the squat*, your abdominal musculature will be heavily
stressed (so will your biceps and most other muscle groups).

maximal poundage per lift). Power training, with maximal weight and low reps, is best left to competitive lifters.

On heavy days, you will attempt to better your last 5 x 5 work weight by five pounds. It matters not if you are bench-pressing 95 lbs. for five sets of five repetitions; the following session you *will* bench 100 lbs. for five sets of five. If you do not succeed in completing the 25 (5 x 5) reps with proper form, do not advance the weight during the next session. Complete the 5 x 5 with 100 lbs., *and then* increase the weight. For deadlifts, increase the weight after you are capable of performing *three* sets of 5 (3 x 5).

At what poundage do you start? This will be a matter of trial and error for novice lifters. **DO NOT** even attempt a 1-rep maximum on any movement unless you are an advanced lifter. If you know your 1-RM however, use 87 percent of that number to determine your 5x5 work set poundage. For everyone else, cautiously progress to a weight that you will allow you to *barely* complete five sets of five repetitions with three minutes of rest between sets. *There is no training to failure.* Your goal is to complete the reps *unassisted.* Only unassisted reps count. These are your "work sets." Sets leading up to your target (work) weight *do not count.* These are considered warm-up sets and are *never* to be neglected. Do not wear yourself out during warm-up however.

4. After you have completed your heavy work, proceed with the *secondary* movement: overhead press if squats were your primary movement, bench press if deadlifts were. Squats are accordingly performed after heavy overhead presses and deadlifts after bench press. These are performed with 90 percent of your previous *successful* 5 x 5 weight (for that particular movement). **Scheme:** three sets of eight (3 x 8) with 60-90 seconds between sets, no longer. These sets are geared towards muscle *hypertrophy*.

Note: The **Strength** sets are geared more towards the neural element of the movement (getting the peripheral nerves to fire optimally in response to increasing weight loads) and will ultimately allow you to handle heavier weight during the hypertrophy sets. Strong does not always equate to size. In this protocol however, you will train to be *both* big and strong.

5. **Auxiliary work** is then performed to further stress the muscles utilized in the *secondary* movement. Utilize the exercises depicted in the figure. Select two movements and perform three sets of eight (3 x 8). Utilize 60-90 second rest intervals as per prior. If you successfully complete the three sets, increase your weight by five pounds during the next session. Obviously it is important to keep accurate records. *Vary* your choice of exercises every workout.

AUXILIARY EXERCISES*
ACCORDING TO SECONDARY MOVEMENT PERFORMED:

Overhead Press	Squat	Bench Press	Deadlift
Lateral raise (db)	Leg extension	Front raise (db)	Biceps curl (bar)
Close-grip bench	Stiff-legged deadlift	Triceps pushdown	Hyperextension***
Upright row/raise	Leg press	Flye (db)	Seated row
Triceps extension	Adductor**	Dip***	Leg curl

db = dumbbell

Note: Exercises in red are not to be done within the same session.

* Seek the advice of an experienced trainer for instruction.

** "Selectorize" machine found in most gyms. It is not just for women!

***Weight can be added as needed.

6. Keep alternating the primary (heavy) movement (lower body and then upper body, lower body then upper body...) and hence the secondary/auxiliary exercises. If done properly, you will train a primary movement (heavy) once every two weeks but you will be training *each* on a weekly basis (as they are all secondary movements as well). Does this make sense? I refer you to the table on the following page.

And the cycle repeats on week 3. Of course if you are novice to the program, there will be some trial and error at the start, because the

ALTERNATING PRIMARY AND SECONDARY EXERCISES

Monday	Tuesday	Wednesday	Thursday	Friday	
Primary: Bench Press **Secondary:** Deadlift **Auxiliary**				**Primary:** Squat **Secondary:** Overhead Press **Auxiliary**	WEEK ONE
Primary: Deadlift **Secondary:** Bench Press **Auxiliary**				**Primary:** Overhead Press **Secondary:** Squat **Auxiliary**	WEEK TWO

secondary movement poundages are based on *previous* performance (and there is none). That's OK. You've got to start somewhere, right? Guestimate and get started! This issue will obviously sort itself out quickly.

Now let's fill in the rest of the grid, starting with the **Strength-Endurance** workouts.

7. Wednesday's **Strength-Endurance** session stresses pull/carry/hold modalities. Very functional strength. The workout is of moderate to high intensity and lasts 30 minutes typically (no longer). The workout should bring your body to the "lactate threshold" (else it is not challenging enough) which ultimately improves glucose tolerance and provides a chelating effect, both of which improve the health of your blood vessels.

There are myriads of potential **Strength-Endurance** workouts. Feel free to design your own, but do not exclude the pull/chin up as this is the foundational movement (a "pillar").

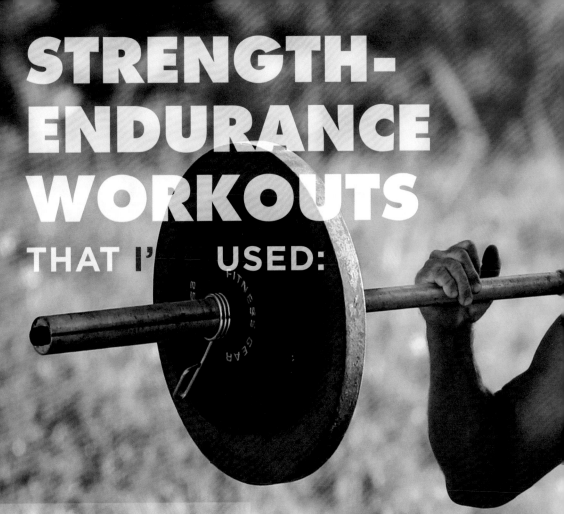

STRENGTH-ENDURANCE WORKOUTS

THAT I'VE USED:

30 MINUTE TIME LIMIT.

This is *not* a race. <u>There are no races when weights are involved</u> (unless you are racing to a local ER having been injured as a result of stupidity). If you are reasonably conditioned, the time constraints will be a non-issue. To make the workouts more difficult as you progress, add weight or chin/pull-up reps. A "strong" individual can do 20 *dead-hang* pull-ups, chest to the bar (no kips and no half reps as, are advocated in the many activity-based protocols out there).

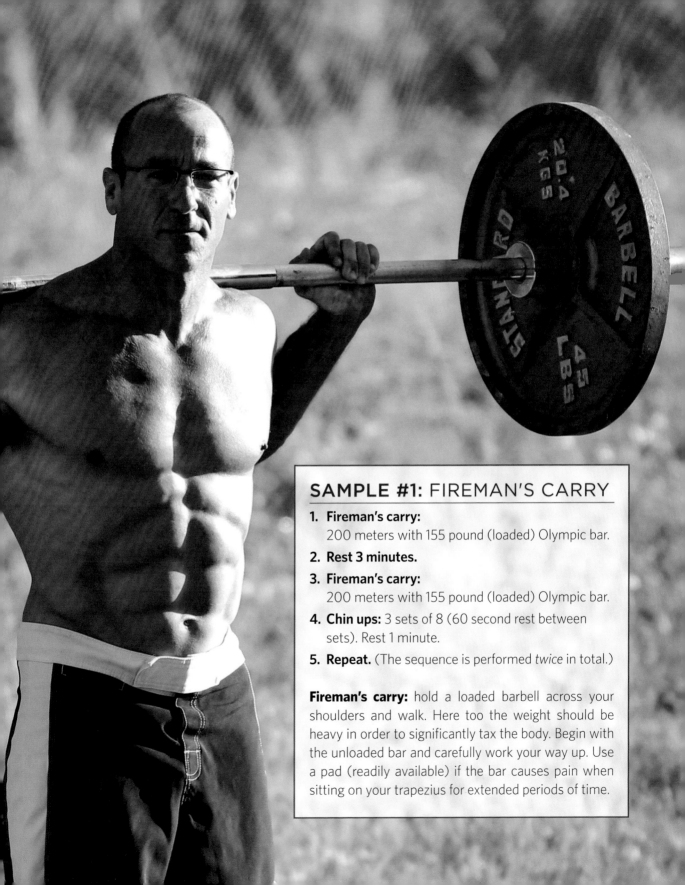

SAMPLE #1: FIREMAN'S CARRY

1. **Fireman's carry:**
   200 meters with 155 pound (loaded) Olympic bar.

2. **Rest 3 minutes.**

3. **Fireman's carry:**
   200 meters with 155 pound (loaded) Olympic bar.

4. **Chin ups:** 3 sets of 8 (60 second rest between sets). Rest 1 minute.

5. **Repeat.** (The sequence is performed *twice* in total.)

Fireman's carry: hold a loaded barbell across your shoulders and walk. Here too the weight should be heavy in order to significantly tax the body. Begin with the unloaded bar and carefully work your way up. Use a pad (readily available) if the bar causes pain when sitting on your trapezius for extended periods of time.

SAMPLE #2: FARMER'S WALK

1. **Farmer's walk:** 200 meters with 45 pound dumbbells.
2. **Rest 3 minutes.**
3. **Farmer's walk:** 200 meters with 45 pound dumbbells.
4. **Pull ups:** 3 sets of 8 (60 second rest between sets).
5. **Repeat.** (The sequence is performed *twice* in total.)

Farmer's walk: walk with dumbbells held at your side. Select a weight that you can hold for at least 2 minutes prior to resting. This will dramatically increase your grip strength over time which will secondarily augment your deadlifting capabilities.

SAMPLE #3: SANDBAG

1. **Sandbag "shouldering":** 15 reps. Rest 1 minute.
2. **Chin up:** 8 reps. Rest 1 minute.
3. **Deadlift:** 135 x 15. Rest 1 minute.
4. **Pull ups:** 8 reps. Rest 1 minute.
5. **Repeat.** (The sequence is performed *three* times in total.)

Sandbag: a staple in any strongman's regimen! There are many exercises that can be performed with a sandbag including basic "shouldering" from a grounded start position (onto alternating shoulders), bear hug walks, presses and curls. The sandbag should weigh *at least 1/3* of your body weight. *Do not* use the straps/handles on the bag as this will maximize the indirect grip (forearm) work. The goal of sandbag training is to expose the body to lifting *heavy, awkward* objects. It is yet another type of varied stimulus to which the body must adapt. This type of training can be brutal and is for the advanced trainee only. As always, utilize proper form: at the start, stay low with your knees bent, body in close approximation to the sandbag. Never let the sandbag fall away from your body as this will predispose you to injury.

SAMPLE #4:

1. **Sprint** for 5 seconds. **Walk** for 55 seconds.
2. At the minute mark, perform 20 **pushups.** Should these need to be performed on your knees (as opposed to standard form), so be it. Your goal is to get through the entire session.
3. **Rest 1 minute.**
4. Turn around and *repeat* the sequence a *total* of 10 times.
5. **Chin up:** 3 sets *to failure.* 2-minute rest between sets.

SAMPLE #5:

1. **Deadlift:** 135 x 10.
2. **Row:** 250m *sprint* (Concept 2 ergometer or similar).
3. **Chin up:** 8 reps.
4. **Row:** 250m *sprint.*
5. **Rest 3 minutes.**
6. **Repeat.** (The sequence is performed *three* times in total.)

SAMPLE #6: RUCKSACK WALK

1. **Rucksack walk:** obtain one from your local Army/Navy store. Place several sand-filled garbage bags (totaling 25 percent of your body weight) into the sack. Shoulder the rucksack (using the straps) and walk .5 miles. Rest 3 minutes.
2. **Chin ups:** 1 set of 10.
3. **Repeat.** Perform the entire sequence *twice*. As you progress, increase the weight until you can safely handle 50 percent of your body weight in the rucksack. Use extreme caution when handling the rucksack particularly if you have had low-back problems in the past. Rucksack walks are not for the fainthearted and are utilized in military training.

Note: These workouts are not set in stone. They are examples of workouts that I have used in the past. Modify them accordingly to suit the available equipment (gym or home setting). As above, *do not exclude the pulling movements.* These workouts are designed to stress hold/pull/carry modalities and will supplement your deadlift and squatting power. Get those lifts up weight-wise and I guarantee you'll be a different human in 6 months! Let's move on...

8. Tuesday and Thursday's **Steady-State Endurance** sessions are straight-forward. Personally, I hate endurance work but it is a necessary evil. Remember you want to have the ability to lift heavy weights (for your size) and run up 10 flights of stairs without being winded. The problem is that it is difficult to do both (as discussed earlier). So we will err on the side of strength development, but still stress the cardiovascular system in isolation twice weekly. To do this, select any of the various modalities: row, walk, run, swim, cycle.

And you don't need any fancy machines. These gadgets are nothing more than hyped-up contraptions with little, if any, physiologic basis or merit. They are a waste of money and are typically sold to the emotionally charged buyer seeking an easy route to six-pack abs. Again, this will never happen *easily*. It takes work. No machine will deliver this to you. So save your money. It's better invested in a gym membership, as opposed to a product which will ultimately double as clothes hanger.

You've chosen to walk. So be it. What we're aiming for is a heart rate 70 percent of your maximal rate (estimated as: 220 – age) sustained for 30 minutes. If you are 40 years old:

$$(220-40) \times .70 = 126 \text{ beats per minute (bpm)} \times 30 \text{ minutes}$$

You will have to walk fast in order to drive your heart rate up to 126 bpm (particularly if you are well-accustomed to endurance work). If this is problematic, you may hold a dumbbell in each hand, curling it as you walk. In response to the additional muscular contractions (of the arm), heart rate will increase (to meet oxygen demands). Limit your endurance work to 30 minutes *at target heart rate*. You otherwise run the risk of stalled progress and size loss (as type IIb fibers will atrophy to allow for expanding capillary beds to serve the type I fibers). People often approach me and ask of my opinion in regards to their failed progress in the gym. My first question is invariably, *"How much running are you doing?"* Get the picture? Get out of the running mode. Else run (no pun intended) the risk of remaining a pipsqueak.

Why is it that I'd see the same people at the gym, year after year, looking exactly the same as they did in years earlier—or even worse? Because someone told them that doing "cardio" day in and day out would confer the most benefit. Or because someone told this physician friend of mine (female) that weight training would make her "bulky." Come on people! Use a little introspection. Has all that "cardio" delivered as promised? Is it providing your body with that much-needed daily challenge? Or that provocative stimulus to which you will adapt and by virtue, improve physically? Doubtful. And that's why you mount the treadmill, day in and day out, having experienced few if any physical gains during the past several years. You've got to start thinking about what you are doing. And why you are doing it. Don't expect results haphazardly going through the motions.

The body wants to accommodate the stress imposed upon it. How does it do this? By getting stronger or becoming a more efficient endurance machine if you will. In this way, energy output is minimized. Therefore, unless you present the body with a different stimulus time after time (through a progressive resistance training program), the body will adapt fairly quickly (i.e. become more efficient at that particular exercise or activity). And therein lies the futility (not utility) of daily running.

Now, filling in the grid:

Monday	Tuesday	Wednesday	Thursday	Friday	
Primary: Bench Press **Secondary:** Deadlift **Auxiliary**	**Steady-State Endurance**	**Strength-Endurance**	**Steady-State Endurance**	**Primary:** Squat **Secondary:** Overhead Press **Auxiliary**	**WEEK ONE**
Primary: Deadlift **Secondary:** Bench Press **Auxiliary**	**Steady-State Endurance**	**Strength-Endurance**	**Steady-State Endurance**	**Primary:** Overhead Press **Secondary:** Squat **Auxiliary**	**WEEK TWO**

And the cycle repeats itself. Again, weekends are *completely off.*

A COUPLE OF ADDITIONAL POINTS

Abdominals are to be worked at the conclusion of *every* session, as a strong midsection is integral to the development of strength and power. Although you may not believe so, all of the trained exercises are heavily reliant on a strong mid-section. The prescribed exercises further condition the abdominal wall post-training. The additional abdominal work is not geared towards your development of a "six-pack." It simply doesn't work that way kiddo.

That said, there is no indication for a separate day of "core" training. There is no need for discrete "core" boot camp sessions. These are simply money-making rackets, targeting the emotionally crazed masses who desire a piece of the latest and greatest. I would just walk away and spend my money elsewhere (educating myself, for example). You see, if you follow the very straightforward protocol outlined above, you will engage the mid-section in a more functional, yet indirect manner. How? By doing the basic exercises. Nothing special. You don't need a complex abdominal regimen to attain your six-pack. I haven't done a sit-up in at least 10 years! And guess what? They're potentially injurious to your low back. Far more important than midsection training is nutrition, if your goal is to attain that ripped look.

If you seek a defined mid-section (which does not necessarily translate to strength), reduce your body fat to fairly low levels. People ask me often if I "do

LEG RAISE

This is an intermediate strength movement for the abdomen (see text). Minimize hip flexor activation by keeping your torso upright (I actually imagine myself leaning forward). Bring the toes past the horizontal plane if possible, attempting to maintain a 'V' position instead of an 'L.' And ditch those silly straps used to suspend the body from the bar. Instead develop the *necessary* grip strength to hold your body weight. These may be performed for repetitions or as a static hold (as was performed here for 45 seconds). **Note:** those boots serve as counter weights which amplify the brutal nature of prolonged static holds.

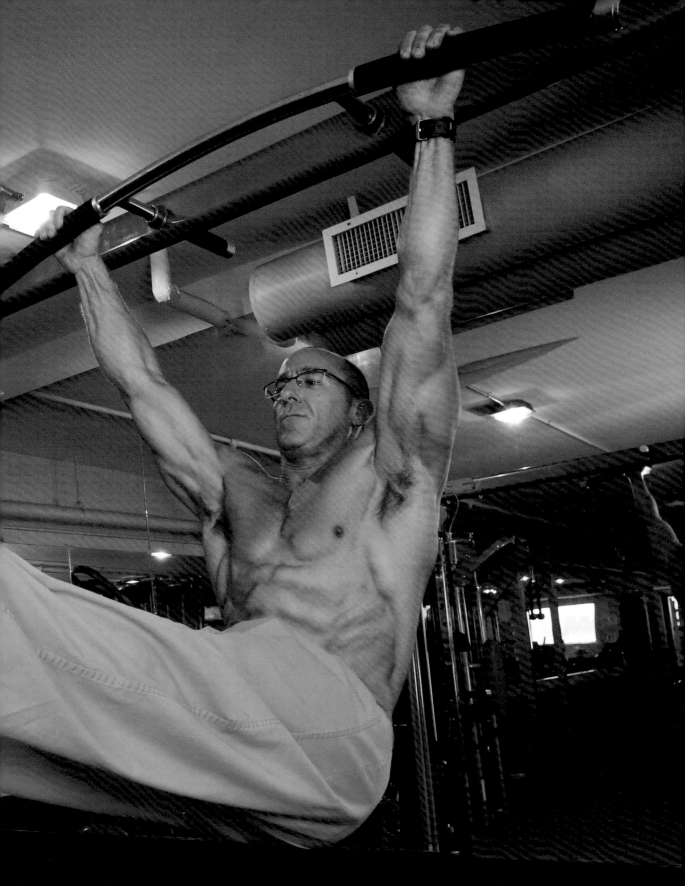

a lot of crunches." I do *none*. But I do work my mid section via the afore-mentioned exercises and maintain a lean physique. *This is the key.* Every-one, yes that includes you, has well-formed abdominal musculature un-derneath that spare tire. Accordingly, you must reduce your body fat to 9 percent or less to unroof that "six-pack." It is there, I promise you. But it is *not* a function of abdominal work. Bodybuilders aspire to have that "ripped" look. Relative to powerlifters, they are *not* strong. They have sacrificed strength (by dieting during competition season) and shed fat in order to build that Adonis-like physique.

Take it from me, a lean midsection has *nothing* to do with the "Ab Blaster," or electronic abdominal belts. These are gimmicks. Don't waste your money. Abs take work, period. *That's why most people don't have them.*

At the conclusion of each workout, I add 3 sets of 15-20 *leg raises.* There are several stages of progression:

a. ***Legs bent:*** beginner

b. ***Legs straight ('L' position):*** intermediate

c. ***Legs straight,* instep to the crossbar (inverted):** for the advanced trainee

Note: Leg raises should be performed with 60-90 second rest intervals (NO longer)

Steady-State Endurance work should, if tolerated, be performed on an empty stomach immediately upon awakening. Why? This will accelerate fat burning as the body is already in a catabolic state (after eight hours of sleep). Remem-ber, the lack of insulin (as in a fasted state) promotes lipolysis or fat burning. Take advantage of this phenomenon and do not consume *any* carbohydrate prior to the training session (this is in stark contrast to pre-resistance train-ing nutrition). Trainees often make this mistake (by drinking a glass of orange juice, for example) and completely shut down the fat-burning process. In the fasted state, the body preferentially utilizes fat as an energy source. Once you drink a glass of orange juice, your body will utilize the consumed glucose to fuel your workout. You will still derive the cardiovascular benefits of the **Steady-State Endurance** session however the lipolytic (fat-burning) effect will be markedly diminished, if not eliminated.

Upon completion of your session wait approximately 30 minutes (to allow for continued fat burning) and then consume a low glycemic index carbohy-drate and protein-laden breakfast.

A word about **nutrition, rest, and stalled progress:** It is imperative that you obtain adequate sleep (8 hours if possible) while engaged in the protocol. Similarly, sound nutrition with particular attention to high protein intake and caloric surplus (exceeding your *sedentary* BMR by approximately 500 kcal daily) is critical. Remember, you are electively traumatizing your muscles and they require substrate for repair. This is precisely why I do not advocate such training programs in the context of a weight loss "diet." It is difficult to lose fat and gain muscle unless you are an advanced trainee and know how to modulate your diet (with caloric cycling). *If your goal is to remain in an anabolic state and pack on muscle,* you must generate a caloric surplus (by eating a lot). Losing fat requires a caloric deficit to allow your body to enter a catabolic state. "Caloric cycling," an advanced protocol, allows one to ride the fine line between anabolism and catabolism. It is *not* easy, requires tremendous discipline, and the "body mindfulness" of an experienced trainee. In addition, if you consistently error on the side of caloric deficit, you will lose both muscle and fat, and your gains will slip or progress stall. There are three main reasons why individuals fail to make progress:

1. **Inadequate or suboptimal nutrition**
2. **Inadequate sleep**
3. **Inadequate training intensity**

In the event that your progress stalls, take a very close look at these three factors. Error on the side of taking an additional day off from training if need be. Don't train if you are ill. If your workday has been extremely stressful and your nutrition poor, consider taking the day off. Rest and eat. Don't bother training if the session will ultimately detract from your progress (by adding stress from which you must recover). *The gym is for productive work only.* Else you are wasting your time.

The last point serves as an excellent segue to my final (and likely most important) one. **Every three months, regardless of how you are feeling, take an entire week off all resistance training.** This will allow the body to recover from not only training-associated stress, but from the cumulative external stresses assumed by each and every one of us. Don't think twice or feel guilty about taking time off. The change (and rest) does the body good. Now reread this paragraph.
Twice.

Get going!
Make next Monday day #1 of the protocol and welcome to a stronger you...

Afterword

As you know by now, I feel no compulsion to beg you, the reader, to listen to me. I don't operate that way, no pun intended. I'd rather speak to you through my actions, by **showing** you the things that have worked for me over the course of many years. Hopefully some of the concepts and ideas have stuck. I am not the fat cardiologist demanding that you lower your fat intake in an effort to lose weight or better your lipid profile. The pictures in this book are not airbrushed, I can assure you. I am living proof that attention to detail, application of nutritional and exercise knowledge, and diligence works. It's just that simple. **There are no magic pills, none.** At least none that will grant you long-term health and longevity. At this point, in the context of current biomedical technology, **it's up to you!** The ball's in your court and certainly not in your doctor's.

Fear not though because you now possess some of the basic knowledge needed to significantly improve your health and well-being. By following the recommendations in this book, you will reclaim your physicality and improve your mental acuity, dramatically. You will be leaner and stronger than you've been in years. And your brain will follow suit. Remember, physical exercise slows the development of neurodegenerative diseases such as Alzheimer's. More simply put, strength training works the mind as well as the body.

But do it now! Don't wait until your first bout of crushing chest pain or symptoms of a stroke before making those much-needed lifestyle changes. You're smarter than that. Empowered. Yes, **YOU!** This book has given you the knowledge to...

Assume control by first identifying your disease risk factors and then making the necessary lifestyle changes to reduce your risk of age-related disease. Read and reread this book. Exhaust all available resources in your quest for wellness. Claim your health. Because you can! This is my charge to you.

And remember, you are not alone in this journey. I am reachable through the various social media platforms and my personal website: www.drbrettosborn.com.

Now, get going and...

Get Serious!

Bibliography

Chapter 1

Anderson G. *Chronic care: making the case for ongoing care.*
Robert Wood Johnson Foundation. February 2010.

Boden WE, O'Rourke RA, Teo KK, Hartigan PM, Maron DJ, Kostuk WJ, et al:
Optimal medical therapy with or without PCI for stable coronary disease.
N Engl J Med. 2007 Apr 12;356(15):1503-16.

Cannon WB: "Voodoo" death. *Am J Public Health.* 2002 Oct;92(10):1593–96.

Chapter 2

Gouni-Berthold I, Krone W, Berthold HK: Vitamin D and cardiovascular
disease. *Curr Vasc Pharmacol.* 2009 July;7(3):414-22.

Peterlik M, Grant WB, Cross HS: Calcium, vitamin D and cancer.
Anticancer Res. 2009 Sep;29(9):3687-98.

Spector, R: *A skeptics view of prevention and treatment of heart disease
and stroke.* Skeptical Inquirer. September/October 2010;34(5):43-49.

Tang BM, Eslick GD, Nowson C, Smith C, Bensoussan A: Use of calcium
or calcium in combination with vitamin D supplementation to prevent
fractures and bone loss in people aged 50 years and older: a meta-analysis.
Lancet. 2007 Aug 25;370(9588):657-66.

Chapter 3

Anand P, Kunnumakara AB, Sundaram C, Harikumar KB, Tharakan ST, Lai OS,
et al: Cancer is a preventable disease that requires major lifestyle changes.
Pharm Res. 2008 Sep;25(9):2097-2116.

Ornish D, Magbanua MJ, Weidner G, Weinberg V, Kemp C, Green C, et al:
Changes in prostate gene expression in men undergoing an intensive nutrition
and lifestyle intervention. *PNAS* June 17, 2008 vol.105 no.24:8369-8374.

Chapter 4

Ang ET, Gomez-Pinilla F: Potential therapeutic effects of exercise to the brain. *Current Medicinal Chemistry.* 2007(14):2564-2571.

Birks J, Grimley EV, Van Dongen M: Ginkgo biloba for cognitive impairment and dementia. *Cochrane Database Syst Rev.* 2002;(4):CD003120.

Bu J, Zu H: Effects of pregnenolone intervention on the cholinergic system *Int J Neurosci.* 2013 Nov 11. [Epub ahead of print]

Dimond SJ, Brouwers EM: Increase in the power of human memory in normal man through the use of drugs. *Psychopharmacology.* 1976 Sep 29;49(3):307-9.

Elsabagh S, Hartley DE, Ali O, Williamson EM, File SE: Differential cognitive effects of ginkgo biloba after acute and chronic treatment in healthy young volunteers. *Psychopharmacology.* May 2005;179(2):437-446.

George MS, Guidotti A, Rubinow D, Pan B, Mikalauskas K, Post RM: CSF neuroactive steroids in affective disorders: pregnenolone, progesterone, and DBI. *Biol Psychiatry.* 1994 May 15;35(10):775-80.

Lamb, SM. *Pathways of the brain: the neurocognitive basis of language.* Amsterdam: John Benjamins Publishing Company, 1999.

Li WL, Cai HH, Wang B, Chen L, Zhou QG, Luo CX, et al: Chronic fluoxetine treatment improves ischemia-induced spatial cognitive deficits through increasing hippocampal neurogenesis after stroke. *J Neurosci Res.* 2009 Jan;87(1):112-22.

Medina, AE: Vinpocetine as a potent anti-inflammatory agent. *Proc Natl Acad Sci USA.* 2010 June 1;107(22):9921-9922.

Pereira AC, Huddleston DE, Brickman AM, Sosunov AA, Hen R, McKhann GM, et al: An in vivo correlate of exercise-induced neurogenesis in the adult dentate gyrus. *Proc Natl Acad Sci.* 2007 Mar 27;104(13):5638-5643.

Trejo F, Nekrassov V, Sitges M: Characterization of vinpocetine effects on DA and DOPAC release in striatal isolated nerve endings. *Brain Res.* 2001 Aug 3;909(1-2):59-67.

Tuszynski MH, U HS, Amaral DG, Gage FH: Nerve growth factor infusion in the primate brain reduces lesion-induced cholinergic neuronal degeneration. *J. Neurosci.* Nov 1990;10(11):3604-3614.

Chapter 5

Baechle T, Earle R. *Essentials of Strength Training and Conditioning.*
Illinois: Human Kinetics, 2008.

Delavier, F. *The Strength Training Anatomy Workout II*. Illinois: Human Kinetics,
2010.

Rippetoe, M. *Starting Strength, third edition.* Texas: The Aasgard Company, 2011.

Zatsiorsky VM, Kraemer WJ. *Science and Practice of Strength Training, second
edition.* Illinois: Human Kinetics, 2006.

Chapter 6

de Lorgeril M, Salen P, Martin JL, Monjaud I, Delaye J, Mamelle N:
Mediterranean diet, traditional risk factors, and the rate of cardiovascular
complications after myocardial infarction: final report of the Lyon Diet Heart
Study. *Circulation.* 1999;99:779-85.

Estruch R, Ros E, Salas-Salvadó J, Covas MI, Corella D, Arós F, et al: Primary
prevention of cardiovascular disease with a Mediterranean diet. *N Engl J Med*
2013;368:1279-1290.

Krauss RM, Blanche PJ, Rawlings RS, Fernstrom HS, Williams PT: Separate
effects of reduced carbohydrate intake and weight loss on atherogenic
dyslipidemia. *Am J Clin Nutr* 2006;83:1025-31.

Nordmann AJ, Suter-Zimmermann K, Bucher HC, Shai I, Tuttle KR, Estruch R,
et al: Meta-analysis comparing Mediterranean to low-fat diets for modification
of cardiovascular risk factors. *Am J Med.* 2011 Sep;124(9):841-51.

Ramsden CE, Zamora D, Leelarthaepin B, Majchrzak-Hong SF, Faurot KR,
Suchindran CM, et al: Use of dietary linoleic acid for secondary prevention of
coronary heart disease and death: evaluation of recovered data from the Sydney
Diet Heart Study and updated meta-analysis. *BMJ.* 2013 Feb 4;346:e8707.

Shepherd J, Blauw GJ, Murphy MB, Bollen EL, Buckley BM, Cobbe SM, et al:
PROSPER study group. PROspective Study of Pravastatin in the Elderly at Risk.
Pravastatin in elderly individuals at risk of vascular disease (PROSPER):
a randomised controlled trial. *Lancet.* 2002 Nov 23;360(9346):1623-30.

Tipton KD, Ferrando AA, Phillips SM, Doyle D Jr, Wolfe RR: Post-exercise net
protein synthesis in human muscle from orally administered amino acids.
Am J Physiol. 1999;276:E628-34.

Wolfe, R: The underappreciated role of muscle in health and disease. *Am J Clin Nutr.* 2006;84:475-82.

Chapter 7

Bowden J, Sinatra S. *The Great Cholesterol Myth*. Massachusetts: Fair Winds Press, 2012.

Gropper S, Smith J, Groff J. *Advanced Nutrition and Human Metabolism, fifth edition.* California: Wadsworth. 2009.

Hu J, La Vecchia C, de Groh M, Negri E, Morrison H, Mery L, et al: Dietary trans fatty acids and cancer risk. *Eur J Cancer Prev.* 2011 Nov;20(6):530-8.

Krauss RM, Blanche PJ, Rawlings RS, Fernstrom HS, Williams PT: Separate effects of reduced carbohydrate intake and weight loss on atherogenic dyslipidemia. *Am J Clin Nutr* 2006;83:1025-31.

Kurzweil R, Grossman R. *Transcend.* New York: Rodale, 2009.

Nordmann AJ, Suter-Zimmermann K, Bucher HC, Shai I, Tuttle KR, Estruch R, et al: Meta-analysis comparing Mediterranean to low-fat diets for modification of cardiovascular risk factors. *Am J Med.* 2011 Sep;124(9):841-51.

Rizzo MR, Barbieri M, Marfella R, Paolisso G: Reduction of oxidative stress and inflammation by blunting daily acute glucose fluctuations in patients with type II diabetes: role of dipeptidyl peptidase-IV inhibition. *Diabetes Care.* 2012 Oct;35(10):2076-82.

Chapter 8

Algra AM, Rothwell PM: Effects of regular aspirin on long-term cancer incidence and metastasis: a systematic comparison of evidence from observational studies versus randomised trials. *Lancet Oncol.* 2012 May;13(5):518-27.

Giovannucci E, Liu Y, Hollis BW, Rimm EB: 25-hydroxyvitamin D and risk of myocardial infarction in men: a prospective study. *Arch Intern Med.* 2008 Jun 9;168(11):1174-80.

Kannel WB: "Implications of Framingham study data for treatment of hypertension: impact of other risk factors." *Frontiers in Hypertension Research.* Springer-Verlag. 1981:17-21.

Klein EA, Thompson IM Jr, Tangen CM, Crowley JJ, Lucia MS, Goodman PJ, et al: Vitamin E and the risk of prostate cancer: the Selenium and Vitamin E Cancer Prevention Trial (SELECT). *JAMA*. 2011 Oct 12;306(14):1549-56.

Li W, Yu J, Liu Y, Huang X, Abumaria N, Zhu Y et al: Elevation of brain magnesium prevents and reverses cognitive deficits and synaptic loss in Alzheimer's disease mouse model. *J Neurosci*. 2013 May 8;33(19):8423-41.

Chapter 9

Bjørnholt JV, Erikssen G, Aaser E, Sandvik L, Nitter-Hauge S, Jervell J, et al: Fasting blood glucose: an underestimated risk factor for cardiovascular death. Results from a 22-year follow-up of healthy nondiabetic men. *Diabetes Care*. 1999 Jan;22(1):45-9.

Stampfer MJ, Hu FB, Manson JE, Rimm EB, Willett WC: Primary Prevention of Coronary Heart Disease in Women through Diet and Lifestyle. *N Engl J Med* 2000;343:16-22.

Tuomilehto J, Lindström J, Eriksson JG, Valle TT, Hämäläinen H, Ilanne-Parikka P, et al: Prevention of type 2 diabetes mellitus by changes in lifestyle among subjects with impaired glucose tolerance. *N Engl J Med* 2001 May 3;344(18):1343-50.

Metabolic Syndrome Sidebar

Ekelund U, Luan J, Sherar LB, Esliger DW, Griew P, Cooper A: Moderate to vigorous physical activity and sedentary time and cardiometabolic risk factors in children and adolescents. *JAMA*. 2012 February 15;307(7):704-712.

Levesque J, Lamarche B: The metabolic syndrome: definitions, prevalence and management. *J Nutrigenet Nutrigenomics* 2008;1:100-108.

Ogden CL, Carroll MD: Prevalence of overweight, obesity, and extreme obesity among adults: United States trends 1960-1962 through 2007–2008. *Centers for Disease Control and Prevention: National Health and Nutrition Examination Survey.* June 2010.

Chapter 10

Rosengren A, Hawken S, Ounpuu S, Sliwa K, Zubaid M, Almahmeed WA, et al: Association of psychosocial risk factors with risk of acute myocardial infarction in 1,119 cases and 13,648 controls from 52 countries (the INTERHEART study): case-control study. *Lancet.* 2004;364:953-962.

Chapter 11

Anderson GL, Limacher M, Assaf AR, Bassford T, Beresford SA, Black H, et al: Effects of conjugated equine estrogen in postmenopausal women with hysterectomy: the Women's Health Initiative randomized controlled trial. *JAMA.* 2004 Apr 14;291(14):1701-12.

Kaur P, Jodhka PK, Underwood WA, Bowles CA, de Fiebre NC, de Fiebre CM, et al: Progesterone increases brain-derived neuroptrophic factor expression and protects against glutamate toxicity in a mitogen-activated protein kinase and phosphoinositide-3 kinase-dependent manner in cerebral cortical explants. *J Neurosci Res.* 2007 Aug 15; 85(11):2441-9.

KEEPS Report: "KEEPS Results Give New Insight Into Hormone Therapy," presented at *North American Menopause Society (NAMS),* October 2012.

Ma J, Huang S, Qin S, You C: *Progesterone for acute traumatic brain injury. Cochrane Database Syst Rev.* 2012 Oct 17;10:CD008409.

Rossouw JE, Anderson GL, Prentice RL, LaCroix AZ, Kooperberg C, Stefanick ML, et al: Risks and benefits of estrogen plus progestin in healthy postmenopausal women: principal results From the Women's Health Initiative randomized controlled trial. *JAMA.* 2002 Jul 17;288(3):321-33.

Get Serious Index

ace-inhibitors, 138-139, 152

acetylcholine, 119

acetaminophen overdose, 127

ACL (anterior cruciate ligament), 27

adaptive response, 42, 91

adipocytokines, 95, 97

adipogenesis, 147

adipose tissue, 94, 95

adrenal gland / adrenal fatigue, 34

Advil, 169

aerobics, 25

AGEs (advanced glycation end-products), 31, 90, 92, 145, 149

aging, 167
  blood sugar role in, 145
  body mass and, 96
  drug supplementation to reduce, 121, 131, 141
  food choices and, 100
  genetic component / gene association, 21, 167
  and hormone decline / replacement, 34, 172
  inflammation role in, 103, 104, 145
  joint stability and, 27
  and memory loss, drugs to treat, 120, 121
  nutrition and, 94
  oxidation / free radicals and, 32, 36
  protein role in, 98
  strength training effects on, 21, 24, 31, 35
  stress and, 110-112

age-related diseases, 5, 7, 10, 12, 13, 92, 129
  hormones and, 169
  metabolic syndrome, 154
  spatial memory loss, 119
  tests for, 159

"alien hand" syndrome, 116

alpha-linolenic acid, 102

ALS, 33

Alzheimer's disease, 10, 19, 32-33, 36, 92, 119
  drugs to treat and prevent, 121, 122, 132
  insulin excess related to, 140
  low in India, using turmeric, 133
  magnesium lack and, 135-136
  and progesterone deficiency, 172

Ambien, 169

American Diabetes Association, 164

American Hteart Association, research, 16-17

amino acids, 94, 95

anabolic response / process / hormones, 40-41, 72, 94, 95, 98

Androgel, 171

androgens / androgenic agents, 25, 44

angiopathy, 10, 11, 154

antacids, 28

antibodies, 35, 96

antigens, 20

antibiotics, 136, 162

anti-inflammatory
  aspirin as, 138
  diet, 109
  effect of exercise, 28-29, 36
  effect of neurotrophins, 119
  omega-3 acids as, 103
  resveratrol as, 128
  statins as, 139
  vitamin D_3 as, 132

antioxidants, 3, 33, 34, 36, 102, 116, 129, 167
  resveratrol as, 128

anti-seizure drugs, 121

apoptosis, 101, 132

arachidonic acid, 103

Aricept, 10, 122

arteries, 116, 117, 118. *See also* atherosclerotic heart disease

arthritis / psoriatic, 3, 92, 107, 154

aspirin, 138, 153, 154
atherogenic
  dyslipidemia, 162
  process, 31, 103, 132, 138, 153
atherosclerotic heart disease / plaque /
    atherosclerosis, 7, 11, 16, 19. *See
    also* insulin
  cholesterol role in, 105, 107
  fat role in, 101, 103, 104
  and glucose tolerance test, 146, 149
  high blood pressure and, 152, 153
  stress and, 111
  sugar role in, 93, 145
  vitamin E benefit, 135
athletes, professional, strength training for,
    29–30
Atkins diet, 93
ATP (adenosine triphosphate), 31, 89, 90,
    91, 95, 96, 97, 144, 147, 164
autoimmune process, 100, 153

back / low-back
  exercises for, 62, 65
  injuries, 28, 54
  pain, 15
bacteria clostridium difficile, 136
bacterial pathogens, 32
barbell, 72
basal metabolic rate (BMR), 25, 43
B-complex vitamins, 134, 137
BDNF (brain-derived nerve factor), 119
bench press, 37, 40, 72, 74
  exercise technique, 76–77
  photos, 73, 74, 75
  pitfalls, 77–78
  safety considerations, 76
beta-blockers, 138–139, 152
beta-oxidation, 95

Bextra, 127
Big Pharma, 10, 11, 106, 108, 126–127
bile, 107
biochemical processes / biochemistry /
    biochemical pathways, 3, 88, 90,
    123, 156
  assessing, 159, 162–163, 164
bio-identical hormone replacement therapy,
    168, 170–172
Biology-Online.org, 17
blood clotting, supplements affecting, 131,
    133, 135
blood pressure
  cuff, 149
  elevated, 5, 36, 138, 143–144, 154. *See
    also* hypertension
  monitoring systolic and diastolic,
    150–151, 154
blood sugar / glucose, 88, 91
  control, 3
  fasting, 145
  and GI, 92
  and insulin resistance, 6
  resistance training to reduce, 31
  stress and, 21, 111
  tracking, 149–150
blood tests, 159, 164
blood vessels
  to heart and brain, 153
  homocysteine and, 163
  peripheral, 153
Blue Sky Therapy, 45
BMI (body mass index), 97
bodybuilders, 25, 43, 46, 89, 96
  and bodybuilding journals, 98
  protein for, 99
body fat, 95
body mass, lean, 30, 93, 96, 97

body weight, 6

Bonds, Barry, 30

bone density, 27–28

brain, 116–117

    anti-inflammatory factors, 119

    atrophy, 119

    blood flow in, 117

    blood sugar in, 164

    blood vessels to, 153

    exercise to enhance, 119–120

    fat percentage in, 100

    cancer / tumors, 18, 19, 92, 112

    complexity, 116

    neurons in, 116, 117

    rewiring, 119

brain games, 120

brain power, 36–37

British Medical Journal article on muscle
    strength, 35

Burns, George, 33

buttocks, exercise for, 63

bypass surgery, 10, 106–107, 118

caloric cycling, 193

caloric restriction (CR), 131

cancer

    age-related, 10, 12

    bladder, 129

    brain, 18, 19

    breast, 5, 16, 17, 18, 148

    colorectal, 18

    curcumin to prevent, 133

    diabetes and, 148

    diet related to, 16

    environmental, 10, 16, 18, 19

    gene-related, 16, 18, 21

    inflammatory component, 19, 32

    insulin related to, 140

liver, 18

lung, 18

    muscular strength and, 35

    obesity and, 30

    ovarian, 18

    prevention, 2, 10, 20

    prostate, 168

    risk factors, 5, 146

    strength training effect on, 36

    trans fats and, 105

    vitamin supplement as protection
        against, 132

Cannon, Dr. Walter, 7

carbohydrates, 89, 90–91

    complex, 91, 147

    in diet, 108, 126

    simple, 90–91, 111

carcinogens, 111, 137

"cardiac caths," 11

cardiologists, 11

cardio-protective, red wine as, 128

cardiovascular system / fitness / disease /
    risk factors, 26, 34, 35, 107, 108

    Framingham Study of mortality, 138

    glucose tolerance and morbidity, 146

catabolic effect / catabolism, 6, 95, 111

catalase, 32

cataracts, 92

cerebrovascular disease, 19, 138, 144

cervical spondylosis, 153

childhood obesity, 11, 157

chin-up / pull-up, 40

    exercise techniques, 82

    photos, 83–84

    pitfalls, 85

    safety considerations, 82

cholesterol, 105–108, 139

    in food versus blood, 106

HDL, 107, 160

hormones and, 173

LDL, 101, 105, 106, 107, 140, 160

chronic

diseases, 13, 21

fatigue, 111

inflammation, 5, 36, 129, 153

stress, 7

cigarette smoking, 36, 134. *See also* tobacco

claudication, 153

cloning

human, 17

sheep, Dolly, 17

cognitive disorders, drugs for, 121

colitis ("C diff"), 136

collagen, 153

connective tissue, 27

CoQ-10, 140

coronary artery disease (CAD) / coronary
    bypass, 7, 11, 16, 32, 90, 105, 106,
    118, 154, 160

coronary heart disease (CHD)

and cholesterol and fats, 106–107, 109

deaths from, 102, 109

diabetes and, 148

Mediterranean diet to prevent, 102

water intake to reduce, 137

corticosteroids, 92

cortisol, 34, 36, 96, 106, 160, 168, 173

Courage Trial, 11

CRP (C-reactive protein,) 28

CRP test, 162

curcumin / curry powder, 129, 133

cycling, 97

cytokines, 20, 36, 92, 149, 154

deadlift, 37, 40, 62, 65, 120, 179

exercise technique, 70

photos, 63, 64, 66, 67, 68, 69

pitfalls, 71

safety considerations, 66

degenerative process, 3

degenerative spine disease, 30

dehydration, 137

Delavier, F., 82

deltoid muscles, 56, 72

dementia. 119. *See also* Alzheimer's

preventing, 2

morbidity and mortality, 36

Deprenyl, 120

DHA (fatty acid), 100

DHEA, 35

diabetes. *See also* type II diabetes

age-related, 10

early onset, 12

epidemic, 88, 149

inflammation and, 92, 103

and insulin as risk factor, 144–145

juvenile (type 1), 91, 144

muscle protein as protector, 96

and omega-3 fatty acid increase, 103

pre-, test for, 146, 148

preventing, 2

diet, 3, 155

American, 104, 111

anti-inflammatory, 109

cancer related to, 16

French, 102

low-fat, 108

Mediterranean, 103, 108

optimal, 36

plant-based, 21

poor, 88

related to genes, 21

dieting, haphazard, 87

disease(s). *See also* age-related diseases;

chronic; heart diseases
  cancer-related, 16
  cerebrovascular, 19, 138, 144
  cholesterol-related, 105–107
  environmental, 10, 16, 18, 19, 126
  gingiva (gum), 103, 162
  inflammatory component of, 19, 20, 30, 31, 32–33, 103, 104, 109
  kidney, 152
  money factor in, 10, 127, 129
  neurodegenerative, 37
  rheumatic, 154
  resistance and regression through exercise, 29, 33
  risks / risk factors, 2, 4, 5, 36, 152, 159
disease prevention, 2–3, 7, 10, 13, 20, 28, 30, 109, 143
DNA, 16, 17
  damage, 31, 32, 132
  methylation, 163
donepezil, 122
drugs, smart, 120–121
drug trials, 127
dyslipidemia, 5, 36, 139

Ecotrin, 138
EGCG in green tea, 132
eicosanoids, 102
elderly. See aging
endarterectomy, 118
endothelium, 92, 93, 107, 161
endurance training / athletes, 35, 95
energy balance, 26
environmental
  diseases, 10, 16, 19, 126
  pollutants / toxins, 16, 18, 20, 129
epigenetics, 21
ergogenic aids, 129

estradiol, 160, 169
estrogen, 106, 168, 171, 173
exercise, 155
  anti-inflammatory effect of, 28–29
  daily, 36, 126
  defense system effect, 33
  hormone effect, 168
  importance of, 3, 5–6
  intensity, 41
  in physical therapy, 29
  as preventive measure, 11, 12
  weight-bearing, 25
exothermic processes, 25–26

Fasting Blood Sugar test, 145, 146, 155
fat, dietary, 89, 106
  bad and good, 88, 100, 101
  saturated and unsaturated, 100–102, 108, 109
  trans, 101
fatty acids, 90, 94, 95
  omega-3 and omega 6, 102–103, 104, 108, 109
FDA, drug regulation by, 13, 126, 127, 128, 129
female. See women
fiber, dietary, 102, 126
fight or flight response, 34
Finnish Diabetes Prevention Study, 149
fish oil, 127, 130
fitness regimens, checking, 44
folic acid, 163
food(s), 89. See also nutrition
  fatty, 93
  good and bad, 4, 12, 41, 89
  labels, 90
  glycemic index, 93
  inflammation preventive, 103, 109

micro and macro-nutrient, 20
    sugary, 88, 94
Framingham Study, 138, 150
free radicals, 3, 19, 20, 31–32, 33, 34, 36,
        129, 167
    cholesterol and, 107, 109. *See also*
        inflammation
    and free radical theory of aging, 31
    long-distance running and release of, 110
    scavengers (NGF and BDNF), 119
French diet, 102
French Paradox, 128
fructose, 90

gene(s) / genome
    blaming, 16, 21
    cholesterol production by, 140
    expression, 18, 21
    food as affecting, 21
    and hepatic synthesis, 106
    and protein synthesis, 41
    resistance training and strength training
        effect on, 21
    as tumor suppressor, 18
    up- and down-regulated, 21
    utilizing, 19
genetic(s)
    aging component, 167
    Alzheimer's predisposition, 36
    code, 17
    methylation defects, disposition, 163
    mutations, 19
    risk factors, 143
    testing, 16
    weight gain, predisposition, 87
genomes, 19, 132, 150
GERD, 125
Gerstmann's syndrome, 116
gingiva (gum) diseases, 103, 162

ginkgo biloba, 121–122
GlaxoSmithKline (GSK), 127, 128
glioblastoma multiforma, 18, 19
glucometer, 145, 146, 154
gluconeogenesis, 95
Glucophage, 140
glucose, 90, 91,163
    for ATP generation, 97, 144
    control, 31
    excess, 88
    fasting test, 145, 146, 155
    homeostasis, 91
    muscle storage of, 96
    as reference food, 92
    tolerance, 30
Glucose Tolerance Test (GTT), 145–148, 155
GLUT receptors, 96
glycation, 31, 36, 92
glycemic index (GI), 92–93, 94
glycogen, 90, 96
goals, setting, 42–43, 44–45
Gravitron™, 85
green tea, 129, 132
growth hormone, 34, 89, 96, 168
gyms, workout, 23, 24, 85, 176

Halfhill, Renée, 45
hamstrings, 63
Harman, Denham, 31
Harvard School of Public Health study, 154
HDL (high density lipoprotein), 105–108
health
    as a choice, 7, 109
    disease-oriented approach to, 2
    good, 4, 88
    as a lifestyle / lifetime endeavor, 27, 37,
        123
    maintenance, 24
healthcare system

costs, 9

and education lack, 11–12

failure of current, 4, 10–11, 13

spending, 13

heart, and blood vessels to, 88 153

heart attacks and heart disease, preventing, 2, 10, 11, 93, 104, 111, 116, 117–118, 119

healthy lifestyle, study, 154

insulin role in, 144–145

ischemic, 138

risk factors, 149, 150

and supplementation, 138, 154

heartburn, 125

hemoglobin A1C test, 163–164

hepatic synthesis, 106

hip, squats for, 47

Hippocrates, 111

HMO's, 11

homeostasis, 26

homocysteine, 134, 163

Homo sapiens, genetic code, 17

hormonal response, 6, 40, 49, 72

hormone(s) / hormone imbalance, 5, 34, 41, 106, 172. *See also* steroid hormone cascade

growth, 35, 89, 96

pancreatic (insulin), 91, 96, 144

steroid, 122, 173

synthetic, 170

testosterone, 34, 35, 41

vitamin D$_3$ as, 132

hormone panels, 165, 170

hormone replacement therapy (HRT), 35, 165, 168–169, 172

bio-identical, 170

hsCRP, 162

human

cloning, therapeutic and reproductive, 17

evolutionary process, 17–18

Hydergine, 120

hydration, optimal, 137

hydrogen peroxide, 32

hyperinsulinemia, 147

hypertension, 5, 137, 138, 139, 140, 143

defined, 151

medications, 152

monitoring, 150–151

prevalence of, 152

systolic and diastolic, 150–151

hypertrophy training, 97

hypoglycemia and hyperglycemia, 91, 145

illness. *See* disease(s)

immune system / response, 20, 21, 35, 111

sleep effect on, 112

vitamin supplements for, 132

immunoglobulins, 96

India, low rate of Alzheimer's disease, 133

inflammation, 3, 5, 20. 36. *See also* Metabolic Syndrome

and aging, 145

arthritis, 92

and atherosclerotic disease, 107

chronic, 20, 36, 129, 153

as cause of disease, 19, 20, 30, 31, 103, 104, 109

sugar and, 88

inflammatory

proteins, 18

response / process, 20, 41

injury prevention, 40

ischemic heart disease, 138

insulin, 41, 89, 90, 91, 96, 140, 144. *See also* diabetes; inflammation; type II diabetes

and heart disease, 93–94

sensitivity, 96, 136

ups and down, 91–92
insulin/IGF-I signaling pathway, 89
insulin-mediated process, 90
insulin resistance (IR), 5, 6, 21, 88, 92, 97,
        100, 111, 143, 144
    and high blood pressure, 154
    and obesity, 152
    tests for, 145, 146–147
insulin sensitivity, 31, 128, 146, 147, 148, 149,
        152, 155
insurance companies, 11
intelligence, smart drugs for, 123
intensity, training, 41–42
INTERHEART study, 160
internet misinformation, 4

Japanese, longevity, 128, 132
joint
    injury, 27
    stability in elderly, 29
Jolie, Angelina, mastectomy, 16
Jones, Arthur, 42
Journal of the American Medical Association
        (JAMA), 157
juvenile diabetes, 91, 144

ketoacidosis, 137, 145
kidney stones / kidney disease, 137, 152
kipping, 85
knee injuries, 27
Kronos Early Estrogen Prevention Study
        (KEEPS), 168

LaLanne, Jack, 41
latissimus dorsi ("lats"), 63, 72, 81
LDL / oxidized LDL (low density
        lipoprotein), 20, 105–108
lean body mass. *See* body mass
Life Extension®, 127, 137

lifestyle
    modification, 21, 149, 155
    sedentary / poor, 21
ligaments, 27
linoleic acid, 109
lipid
    peroxidation, 132
    profile, 140, 159, 160–161
Lipitor, 106
lipolysis, 95
lipoproteins, 161
liver, and liver failure, 106, 107, 127
lockout position, 73, 75
longevity, cardiovascular health and, 36
lordosis, lumbar, 53, 54, 66
Lou Gehrig's Disease (ALS), 33
Lovaza, 127
low-back. *See* back
lupus, 153
Lyon Diet Heart Study, 102

magnesium and magnesium deficiency,
        135–136
McGuire, Mark, 30
Medicare, 13
meditation, 112
Mediterranean diet, 102, 108
memory loss
    age-associated, 119, 120
    omega-3 fatty acids to offset, 128
Metabolic Syndrome, 5, 6, 12, 21, 105, 111,
        152, 154, 155, 156–157, 162
metabolism, boosting, 25, 97
metabolites, 107
metaformin, 140–141, 148, 154
methylation, 134, 163
Mevacor, 106
Michaels, Brett, 110
micronutrients, 98, 129, 137

mitochondria, 31

monitoring, self-, 143, 144

motor function, metabolic role of, 96

multiple sclerosis, 100, 153

multivatims, 137

muscle(s), 27, 63, 95

    abdominal, 189

    biceps, 81

    damage, exercise-induced, 20

    exercise, 24–26

    fast-twitch fibers, 97

    glucose in, 147

    hypertrophy, 35

    injury, 41

    leg, 190

    lumbar, 65

    magazines, 176

    protein, 95–96

    skeletal, 24, 97

    soreness, 40

muscle fiber types, 176

muscle mass, 6, 21, 35, 97, 111

muscular hypertrophy, 25, 26

musculoskeletal system, 26, 27

mutation, 18

    BRCA, 16

    p53, 18, 19

myalgias, 139

myelin and myelin sheath, 100, 106

MVPA (moderate-to-vigorous-intensity physical activity), 12, 157

myocardial infarction, 153. *See also* heart attacks

myocyte, 97

Namenda, 10

National Academy of Sciences, 21

National Health and Nutrition Examination Survey of obesity, 157

National Osteoporosis Foundation, 28

National Science Foundation, 29

natural selection, 117

Nautilus, Inc., 42

nerve growth factor (NGF), 119

neurodegenerative diseases / process, 37, 119, 121, 132

neuro-enhancer, 121

neurogenesis / 36–37, 120

neuromuscular efficiency / integrity, 25, 29

neuromuscular stimulus, 42

neurons / neuronal circuits / pathways, in brain, 116–117, 119

neurosurgery, 1, 6

neurotransmitters, 111–112, 120, 121, 163

neurotrophins, 119

New York City Board of Health ban on trans fats, 105

NGF (nerve growth), 119

nootropids, 120

Nootropil, 121

norepinephrine, 96

nutrigenomics, 21

nutrition / nutrients, 89, 147

    poor, 20, 36, 149

    sound / good, 11, 43, 88, 102, 148, 156, 167

    and strength training, 193

nutritional supplements. *See* supplements

obesity, 4

    childhood, 11, 157

    diabetes association with, 30, 97

    epidemic, 88, 149

    exercise to reduce, 156

    food contributors to, 100–101

    gene association / genetic predisposition, 21, 30–31

    hypertension and, 152

insulin resistance and, 152
    as risk factor, 5
    sleep lack as factor, 43
olive oil, 108
Olympic bar, 50, 58
omega-3 fatty acids, 100, 101, 102–103, 104
    supplements, 127–128, 130–131, 153
omega-6 fatty acids, 101, 103, 104
omega-6:omega-3 ratio, 104
Ornish, Dr. Dean, 21
osteoporosis, 12, 28, 168
overhead press, 40, 57–58
    exercise technique, 61
    photos, 56, 59, 60
    pitfalls, 61
overtraining, 34, 42, 43
oxidation, 31, 32
oxidative stress, 107

pancreas, 90, 91, 144, 147
Parkinson's disease, 36, 119
pathophysiologic process, 153
Pauling, Linus, 126, 134
pectoralis, 56
pelvic musculature, squats for, 47
percutaneous procedures, 11
peripheral arterial disease (PAD), 152, 153, 154
pesticides, 111, 129
pharmaceutical companies / drugs, 10–11, 13, 127, 139. *See also* Big Pharma
phospholipids, 104
physical education in schools, de-emphasis on, 12, 157
physical fitness / activity, 12, 27
physical inactivity as risk factor, 36–37
physical therapy, exercise in, 29
piperine, 133

Piracetam, 121
post-partum depression, 172
powerlifter style, 69
PPO, 11
pre-diabetes. *See* diabetes
pregnenolone, 122
Presidential Fitness Awards, 12
prevention, 116, 118, 143, 159. *See also* disease prevention; injury prevention
probiotics, 136
progestins, 170
progesterone, 160, 168, 169, 172
progress, charting, 42
progressive overload, 26
PROSPER trial, 106
prostate gland, 21, 169
protein(s), body. 35
    AGEs, 30
    contractile (actin and myosin), 97
    inflammatory, 18
    insulin as, 40
    muscle, 95–96
protein, dietary, 89, 94–95, 98–99
    best sources, 99
protein synthesis, 41
Prozac, 120, 169
pull-up and chin-up, 78–79, 81
    photos, 80
    pitfalls, 85

quadriceps, 63, 66, 67, 71
quit — never, 44

RDA
    protein levels, 98
    for Vitamin D, 164
rehabilitation, strength training for, 29

radiation effects, 16

rectus abdominis, 81

red wine, as antioxidant, 102, 128. *See also* resveratrol

Reliant Pharmaceuticals, 127

resistance training, 3, 21, 25, 28, 34
  glucose role in, 97
  growth hormone production in response to, 89
  for protection against disease, 30, 3, 36, 147, 148
  protein for, 98
  for testosterone production, 41

resveratrol, 127, 128
  supplementation, 131–132

rhomboids, 81

Rippetoe, Mark, 51

risk factors, 152, 155. *See also* disease(s); monitoring
  and "after the fact" approach, 10
  cardiometabolic, 12
  exercise, lack of, 6
  modifiable, 2, 5
  testing for, 5

ROS (reactive oxygen species), 33, 36

rotator cuff, 77

round-back lifting, 71

rowing, 40, 97

running / long-distance running, 31, 34, 110

Sacks, Oliver, 116

safety first, 45

salt, sensitivity, 150

sarcopenia, 110

scurvy, 98

SELECT study, 135

self-monitoring, 144

serum glucose, 91–92, 94, 97, 163

serum inflammatory markers, 159

Sirtris Pharmaceuticals, 128

skeletal muscle, 24, 97

sleep, 176
  adequate, importance of, 43, 168
  brain re-boot during, 111
  trackers, 154

smart drugs, 120–123

sodium in diet, 126

soybean oil, 103

soy milk, 99

spine / spinal column
  disorders, preventing, 2, 3
  lumbar, 53
  operations by author, 15, 49
  strengthening, 28

spotter, 50, 76

sprinting, 31

squat, 35, 37, 49, 119, 120, 179, 180
  exercise technique, 50–51
  photos, 46–48, 52, 54, 55
  pitfalls, 53
  safety considerations, 50
  warm-ups, 50

Stairmasters™, 24

starches, 90

statins, 106–108, 139–140

steady-state endurance, 192–193

stenotic arteries / stenosis / stent, 11, 153

steroid hormone cascade, 173

steroids / steroid hormones, 25, 92, 122

strength-endurance workouts, 184
  Farmer's Walk, 186
  Fireman's Carry, 185
  Leg raise, 191–192
  Rucksack Walk, 187–188
  Sandbag, 186

strength training, 23, 24, 34

antioxidant capacity, 33
effect on gene expression, 21
effect on mortality, 36
for musculoskelal system and low back, 27–28
for professional athletes, 29–30
as rehabilitative modality, 29
protocol, 174, 177–179
workouts, 184
stress
cancer related to, 16
chronic, 7
damaging effects of, 110, 168
long-distance running and, 111
muscle protein and, 96
oxidative, 129
response to, 6, 20
psychological, 6, 21, 111
reduction, 11, 118, 147, 148
and stressors, 111–112
stress response, 7
strokes
causes and risk factors, 5, 36, 111, 144, 149
drugs for, 121–122
mortality from, 143
prevention, 2, 116, 117–118, 127
sucrose, 90, 91
sugar, blood. See blood sugar
sugar/insulin interaction, 148–149
sugar, table / refined, 90, 92, 94, 100, 102, 103, 149
superoxide dismutase enzymes, 32
supplements, nutritional, 12, 13, 123, 125–126
vitamin D, 164–165
Sydney Diet Heart Study, 108–109
synapses, 119

Syndrome X. See Metabolic Syndrome

tea. See green tea
tendons, 27, 28
testosterone, 34, 35 34, 35, 41, 106, 107, 160, 168, 169, 173
oral, 171
TMG (trimethylgycine), 163
tobacco / cigarettes
effects of, 20, 112
related deaths, 16
smoke, 33, 107, 111
tocopherols and tocotrienols, 135
toxins / pesticides, 129
training intensity, 41–42
trans fats / trans fatty acids, 101, 104–105
trapezius, 63
treatment versus prevention, 11
triceps, 56, 72
triglycerides / triglyceride synthesis, 93–94, 106
triglyceride:HDL ratio, 106, 161
tumorigenesis, 20, 132
Tylenol, 127
type II diabetes, 5, 9, 10, 21
body fat and, 95
Glucose Tolerance Test to determine, 146–148, 149
insulin resistance leading to, 96, 140, 145
metabolic syndrome and, 154
resistance training to prevent, 30–31
resveratrol supplementation for, 131
sugary foods related to, 88
trans fats and, 105

ultrasound test, 118
urinary tract infections, 137

UV (ultraviolet) radiation, 18, 20, 32

Valsalva maneuver, 51, 66
VAP test, 160, 161–162
vascular disease / vascular endothelium, 12, 103, 107, 117, 118, 134, 141, 143, 145, *See also* diabetes
    hypertension and, 153
    supplements for, 153–154
    tests to indicate risk, 146
vasodilator, hyperglycemia as, 149
vegetable oil, 105, 108
vegetarians, protein foods for, 99
Vinpocetine, 121
Vioxx, 10, 127
vitamins, and tests for
    B-complex / B6 / B12, 134, 163
    C, 126, 129, 134
    D, 5, 12
    D_3, 132–133, 164–165
    E, 135
"voodoo" death, 7

walking, 26–27
warm-ups, 50, 58, 66
warfarin, 28, 135
water intake, importance of, 126, 137
weight belt, 49, 66
weight loss and gain, 3, 7, 93, 111
weight lifting, 35
weights, 23
weight training, 24–26
white blood cells, 31, 153
Wii Fit, 12
wine. *See* resveratrol
women
    chin-ups for, 45
    hormones / HRT / hormone panels, 168

    pull-ups for, 81
    regimented training for, 44
    squats for, 49
    weight training for, 25
Women's Health Initiative (WHI) study, 168
Woods, Tiger, 29–30
workout goal, 24
wound healing and repair, 20
wrist curls, 40

zinc, 163
yoga, 112
yogurt, 136

Zumba™, 24